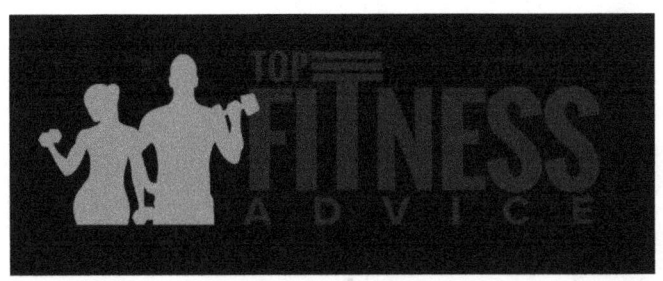

JUICING

5th Edition

The 7-Day Juicing Plan Designed For Weight Loss And To Cleanse & Detox Your Body (Includes Juice Meal Plan & Recipes)

LINDA WESTWOOD

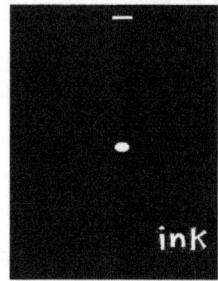

First published in 2015 by Venture Ink Publishing

Copyright © Top Fitness Advice 2019

All rights reserved.

No part of this book may be reproduced in any form without permission in writing from the author. No part of this publication may be reproduced or transmitted in any form or by any means, mechanic, electronic, photocopying, recording, by any storage or retrieval system, or transmitted by email without the permission in writing from the author and publisher.

Requests to the publisher for permission should be addressed to publishing@ventureink.co

For more information about the contents of this book or questions to the author, please contact Linda Westwood at linda@topfitnessadvice.com

Disclaimer

This book provides wellness management information in an informative and educational manner only, with information that is general in nature and that is not specific to you, the reader. The contents of this book are intended to assist you and other readers in your personal wellness efforts. Consult your physician regarding the applicability of any information provided in this book to you.

Nothing in this book should be construed as personal advice or diagnosis, and must not be used in this manner. The information provided about conditions is general in nature. This information does not cover all possible uses, actions, precautions, side-effects, or interactions of medicines, or medical procedures. The information in this book should not be considered as complete and does not cover all diseases, ailments, physical conditions, or their treatment.

You should consult with your physician before beginning any exercise, weight loss, or health care program. This book should not be used in place of a call or visit to a competent health-care professional. You should consult a health care professional before adopting any of the suggestions in this book or before drawing inferences from it.

Any decision regarding treatment and medication for your condition should be made with the advice and consultation of a qualified health care professional. If you have, or suspect you have, a health-care problem, then you should immediately contact a qualified health care professional for treatment.

No Warranties: The author and publisher don't guarantee or warrant the quality, accuracy, completeness, timeliness, appropriateness or suitability of the information in this book, or of any product or services referenced in this book.

The information in this book is provided on an "as is" basis and the author and publisher make no representations or warranties of any kind with respect to this information. This book may contain inaccuracies, typographical errors, or other errors.

Liability Disclaimer: The publisher, author, and other parties involved in the creation, production, provision of information, or delivery of this book specifically disclaim any responsibility, and shall not be held liable for any damages, claims, injuries, losses, liabilities, costs, or obligations including any direct, indirect, special, incidental, or consequences damages (collectively known as "Damages") whatsoever and howsoever caused, arising out of, or in connection with the use or misuse of the site and the information contained within it, whether such Damages arise in contract, tort, negligence, equity, statute law, or by way of other legal theory.

Table of Contents

Disclaimer	3
Who is this book for?	9
What will this book teach you?	11
Chapter 1: What Is The 7-Day Weight Loss Juice?	13
Chapter 2: Why Juice to Lose Weight?	37
Chapter 3: Getting Prepared	57
Shopping List	69
Chapter 4: How to Do the 7-Day Weight Loss Juice	71
Chapter 5: Top Tips for Success	77
Chapter 6: Continue Losing Weight After the Juice	91
Chapter 7: Weight Loss Boosting Secrets	107
Chapter 8: Breakfast Juice Recipes	111
Chapter 9: Lunch Juice Recipes	131
Chapter 10: Dinner Juice Recipes	149
Chapter 11: Snack Juices	177
Conclusion	189
Final Words	191

Would you prefer to listen to my book, rather than read it?

Download the audiobook version for free!

If you go to the special link below and sign up to Audible as a new customer, you can get the audiobook version of my book completely free.

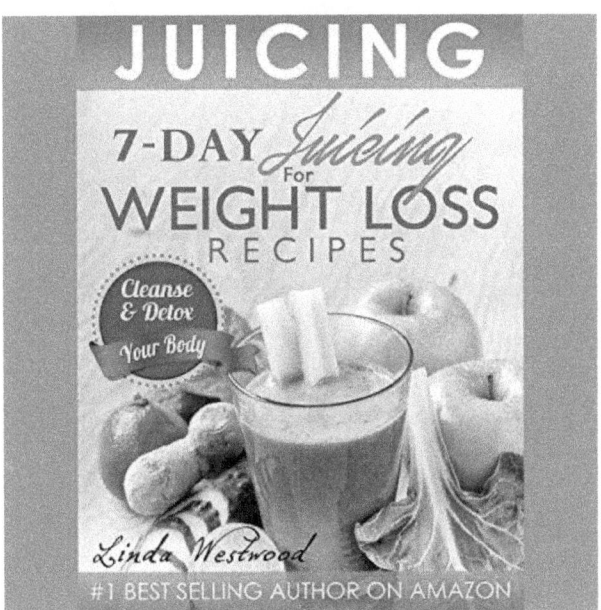

Go here to get your audiobook version for free:

TopFitnessAdvice.com/go/Juicing

Who is this book for?

Are you feeling tired and unhealthy lately?

Do you need to give your weight loss a *good* kick-start?

Do you ever wish you could just melt your belly fat *without even trying?*

Then this book is for you!

I am going to share with you one of the MOST effective juice fasts to completely cleanse your body from the inside out!

I have put it all together a full 7-day Weight Loss Juice plan, along with all the recipes that you need to lose up to 14 pounds in just 7 days!

The best part about this is that you don't even have to do any exercise!

You can be a complete beginner or someone who works out regularly, it doesn't matter!

If this sounds like it could help you, then keep reading...

What will this book teach you?

Inside, I will teach you this 7-day Weight Loss Juice plan that will not only boost your weight loss, but also clear both your mind and body!

You will feel the healthiest you have ever felt – have the most energy you have ever had – and the fat will be melting *effortlessly!*

How? Because you're going to consume a very healthy juice plan that specifically plans out when your body needs certain nutrients – and then gives them to you in those juice recipes.

In this book, I give you the plan right in front of you that will change your life – all you have to do is follow it!

One of the most important things for you to realize when reading this book is that this juice fast *really does work!*

However…

For you to achieve *real success*, you HAVE to apply them to your life.

This is where most people fail – they read through the entire book but do nothing. You MUST try your best to apply as you read through the book!

Chapter 1

What Is The 7-Day Weight Loss Juice?

Welcome to an exciting new chapter, both in this book and in your life.

The 7-Day Weight Loss Juice is an easy-to-follow, super-healthy, enjoyable and effective way to lose weight in just one week.

It will give you a huge boost of vitamins and other nutrients; all while the pounds rapidly drop off, leaving you in superb shape.

The 7-Day Weight Loss Juice is not a fad, or a 'miracle' cure. It is a scientifically sound, nutritionally beneficial, practical and fast acting way to shed unwanted weight at the same time as turbo-charging your health.

So, what's the secret?

What is Juicing?

Juicing is a term that is becoming increasingly popular – and with good reason. Quite simply, it means extracting the juice from ordinary fruits and vegetables and drinking it, with outstanding health and weight-loss benefits.

At its heart, juicing is a simple, highly effective way of extracting the most goodness from nature's best foods. Essentially, you are gaining the intensely nutritive and delicious essences of fruits or vegetables, without chewing and crunching your way through the pounds and pounds of foods you would need to eat to gain the same benefits.

Easy on the digestion and excellent for rapid absorption, fresh juices are a totally natural gift to those who want to stay slim and healthy.

Don't mistake real fresh juice for the high-sugar stuff you get in cartons, let alone the 'juice drinks' with added sugar and heaven knows what else.

Real juice is made straight from the natural ingredients and is best drunk as soon as possible – no artificial additives, no sitting on supermarket shelves for weeks. Real juice is not a miracle cure but it is a wonder-food, one with infinite variations. Plus, when you learn about its amazing nutritional and weight loss potential of the best juices, then you will never look back.

Why is Juicing Good for Us?

Many people have never tried real juice. As you will discover, the fact that we don't make the most of the abundant fruit and vegetables on this planet is a large part of the reason that, according to the World Health Organization, as of 2008, 35% of adults aged 20 and over were overweight, and 11% were obese.

The bad news is that the problem is getting worse... but the really great news is that the solution is all around us.

It is hanging from every fruit tree, growing on bushes and springing up from the soil. It does not require exceptionally expensive equipment or specialized techniques. It just needs a desire to lose weight and a willingness to embrace the juicing lifestyle for just 7 days!

A real juice can be seen as an intense, delicious, flavoursome burst of nutrients, straight from the fruit or vegetables, in liquid form.

But what do they contain? Well, it is no secret that fruit juices contain far more natural sugar than vegetable juices. While some natural sugar is fine, in order to promote weight loss, it is best to keep proportions to 80% vegetable juice, 20% fruit juice.

Isn't Too Much Juice Unhealthy?

There is a misleading modern rumor in some circles that juicing is unhealthy and can even cause you to put on weight. Some even assert that it will lead to diabetes!

So, first of all, let's get a few things straight.

It is certainly true that the average fruit juice causes a rapid rise in blood sugar. This is not the same as when you take a large bite of chocolate, for example, due to the type of naturally occurring sugar in the fruit.

A healthy person would not be adversely affected as they can easily digest and absorb the fruit sugar. This means that the average healthy person will not get diabetes from drinking fruit juice.

Nor will you gain weight – obesity and diabetes are caused by unhealthy diets which mean your body cannot function as efficiently as it should; this simply does not apply to fresh juices.

However, some people suffer from certain conditions, which means it is inadvisable for them to drink fruit juices.

If you are even borderline diabetic, or suffering from candidiasis, or are prone to suffer from thrush, you should refrain from consuming fruit juices.

If you suspect that you may have a yeast infection in the digestive tract, or a low blood sugar level (hypoglycemia), or if you tend to put on weight very easily you need to get professional advice.

If in doubt, please do consult your doctor before embarking on the 7-Day Weight Loss Juice fast.

It should be stated at this point that some people have used low-calorie fasts to actually reverse their diabetes, but this should not be attempted without medical advice.

People who need to watch their sugar intake may still be able to juice, but should just stick to the vegetable juices.

Vegetable juicing, when done correctly, however, would not necessarily pose a medical problem in these cases. There are so many green juice blends that you can try in the 7-Day Weight Loss Juice, all of them are bursting with nutrients and all of them taste delicious.

Plus, green juices have many proven health benefits. You may have been told many times as a child to 'eat your greens' – this is just a palatable way of drinking them and getting an intense hit of their natural goodness.

Fresh green juices such as the ones described in this book may go a long way to improve your blood and health condition.

Read on to learn more about some of the major nutrients contained in a dazzling array of fruit and vegetables.

Which Fruits and Vegetables are Best?

Whatever the juice, provided it comes from fresh, natural produce, it is likely to be bursting with vitamins.

Here are some of the essential nutrients found in fruits and vegetables and their richest natural sources:

Vitamin A

Essential for cell reproduction, stimulating immunity and hormone formation. Supports vision, promotes bone growth, aids tooth development and supports healthy skin, hair, and mucous membranes.

Fruits

- Grapefruit
- Guava
- Mango
- Melon
- Papaya
- Passion fruit
- Tomatoes
- Watermelon

Vegetables

- Bok Choy
- Broccoli
- Brussels Sprouts
- Butternut Squash
- Carrots
- Chinese Broccoli and Cabbage
- Kale
- Leeks
- Peas
- Pumpkin
- Spinach
- Squash
- Sweet Potato
- Swiss Chard

Vitamin B1/Thiamine

Important for energy production and essential for a healthy heart, muscles, and nervous system.

Vegetables

- Asparagus
- Brussels Sprouts
- Butternut Squash
- Green Beans
- Lima Beans
- Okra
- Parsnips
- Peas
- Potatoes
- Spirulina
- Sweetcorn
- Sweet Potato

Fruits

- Avocado
- Breadfruit
- Custard Apple
- Dates
- Grapes
- Grapefruit
- Guava
- Loganberries
- Mango
- Orange
- Pineapple

- Pomegranate
- Watermelon

Vitamin B2/ Riboflavin

Promotes growth, reproduction and red blood cell production, as well as the efficient processing of carbohydrates.

Vegetables

- Artichoke
- Asparagus
- Bok Choy
- Brussels Sprouts
- Chinese Broccoli
- Green Beans
- Lima Beans
- Mushrooms
- Peas
- Pumpkin
- Spirulina
- Squash
- Sweet Potato
- Swiss Chard

Fruits

- Avocado
- Banana
- Custard Apple
- Dates

- Grapes
- Lychee
- Mango
- Mulberries
- Passion Fruit
- Pomegranate
- Prickly Pear

Vitamin B3/Niacin

Powerfully aids the functioning of the digestive system, skin, and nerves, plus it helps convert food to energy.

Vegetables

- Artichoke
- Butternut Squash
- Mushrooms
- Okra
- Parsnip
- Peas
- Potatoes
- Pumpkin
- Spirulina
- Spaghetti Squash
- Sweetcorn
- Sweet Potato
- Winter Squash

Fruits

- Avocado
- Breadfruit
- Custard Apple
- Dates
- Guava
- Loganberries
- Lychee
- Mango
- Nectarine
- Passion Fruit
- Peach

Vitamin B5/Pantothenic Acid

Pantothenic acid is vital, helping us metabolise of food, form hormones and bolster our good cholesterol.

Vegetables

- Broccoli
- Brussels Sprouts
- Butternut Squash
- Green Beans
- Mushrooms
- Okra
- Parsnip
- Potatoes
- Pumpkin
- Spirulina
- Spaghetti Squash
- Squash

- Sweetcorn
- Sweet Potato

Fruits

- Avocado
- Blackcurrants
- Breadfruit
- Custard Apple
- Dates
- Gooseberries
- Grapefruit
- Guava
- Pomegranate
- Raspberries
- Star fruit
- Watermelon

Vitamin B6/Pyridoxine

B6 assists with the creation of antibodies in the immune system. It maintains nerve function, protein action and helps form red blood cells.

Vegetables

- Bok Choy
- Broccoli
- Brussels Sprouts
- Butternut Squash
- Celeriac

- Green Beans
- Green Pepper
- Kale
- Lima Beans
- Okra
- Peas
- Potatoes
- Spirulina
- Spaghetti Squash
- Squash
- Sweetcorn
- Sweet Potato
- Taro root

Fruits

- Avocado
- Banana
- Breadfruit
- Custard Apple
- Dates
- Gooseberries
- Grapes
- Guava
- Lychee
- Mango
- Passion Fruit
- Pineapple
- Pomegranate
- Watermelon

Vitamin B9/Folate

Folate occurs naturally in fresh foods (folic acid is synthetic and found in supplements). Folate is used to produce red blood cells, create DNA and support the nervous system.

It is essential for embryonic development, so it is especially important for pregnant women.

Vegetables

- Artichoke
- Asparagus
- Beetroot
- Bok Choy
- Broccoli
- Brussels Sprouts
- Chinese Broccoli and Cabbage
- Green Beans
- Lima Beans
- Okra
- Parsnip
- Peas
- Potatoes
- Spinach
- Spirulina
- Squash

Fruits

- Avocado

- Blackberries
- Breadfruit
- Custard Apple
- Dates
- Guava
- Loganberries
- Lychee
- Mango
- Orange
- Papaya
- Passion fruit
- Pineapple
- Pomegranate
- Raspberries
- Strawberries

Vitamin C

Vitamin C is an enormously important vitamin. It is an antioxidant, protecting cells against free radicals, which may contribute to cardiovascular disease and cancer.

Vitamin C also has antiviral properties.

Vegetables

- Bok Choy
- Broccoli
- Brussels Sprouts
- Butternut Squash
- Green Pepper

- Kale
- Swiss Chard

Fruits

- Blackcurrants
- Breadfruit
- Grapefruit
- Guava
- Kiwi
- Lychee
- Mango
- Mulberries
- Orange
- Papaya
- Passion fruit
- Pineapple
- Strawberries

Vitamin D

Vitamin D is primarily obtained when the body manufactures it after being exposed to sunshine. It promotes absorption of calcium and magnesium, which are essential for healthy teeth and bones.

Vegetables

- Mushrooms

Vitamin E

Vitamin E is another antioxidant, protecting the body from oxidative damage. It helps form red blood cells and maximizes the benefits of vitamin K.

It can also help heal minor wounds.

Vegetables

- Butternut Squash
- Parsnip
- Potatoes
- Pumpkin
- Spirulina
- Swiss chard
- Taro

Fruits

- Avocado
- Blackberries
- Blackcurrants
- Blueberries
- Breadfruit
- Cranberries
- Guava
- Kiwi
- Loganberries
- Mango
- Mulberries

- Nectarine
- Papaya
- Peach
- Pomegranate
- Raspberries

Vitamin K

Vitamin K is vital to blood clotting, regulating blood calcium levels and maintaining bone health.

Vegetables

- Alfalfa (sprouted)
- Artichoke
- Asparagus
- Bok Choy
- Broccoli
- Brussels Sprouts
- Cabbage
- Carrots
- Cauliflower
- Celery
- Chinese Broccoli
- Cucumber
- Kale
- Leeks
- Okra
- Peas
- Spinach
- Spirulina

- Squash
- Swiss Chard

Fruits

- Avocado
- Blackberries
- Blueberries
- Cranberries
- Grapes
- Kiwi
- Loganberries
- Mango
- Mulberries
- Pear
- Plum
- Pomegranate
- Raspberries
- Tomatoes

So, there you have it – everyday, delicious fruits and vegetables containing an Aladdin's cave of vital nutrients. But we already knew that deep down.

What juicing does is help deliver these nutrients freshly, in substantial quantities and in easily digestible form. High doses of nutrients, relative low amounts of calories, especially in the vegetable juices which naturally contain less sugar.

But why not just eat fruit and veg, you may ask? Why bother to juice everything in the first place? The truth is simple, as it so often is.

Can you imagine trying to munch through six large kale leaves, two carrots, an apple, a handful of spirulina, a whole cucumber and half a lime – just for breakfast? You would have a huge hit of vitamins, but it would take ages, you would also probably get indigestion… and feel pretty sick too.

Juicing the ingredients by putting them into a juicing machine ensures that you benefit from all of the nutrients, with none of the downsides.

But what about all that fiber – isn't that really good for you? Yes!

But when you juice fruit and vegetable – *a lot of fiber is still there!*

Just to be clear, there are two types of fiber in fruit and vegetables – soluble and insoluble fiber:

Soluble Fiber

Soluble fiber is absorbent, much like a sponge. It enhances good bacterial growth, supports digestive health, regulates blood sugar control, lowers blood cholesterol and goes a long way towards giving you that full feeling.

Happily, juices – especially those with passion fruit, avocado, onions, apples and strawberries, amongst others - contain plenty of soluble fiber.

Insoluble Fiber

Insoluble fiber brushes the intestine, speeds up the digestion of food, adds bulk to the stool and keeps you 'regular'. Some of this is removed in juicing although it is still present in smaller amounts.

Also, some people choose to add a little pulp to their juice to bulk it up with natural fiber, others prefer just the purest liquid to ensure the best absorption of nutrients - the choice is yours!

7 Days to a Super New You

So, why does this juicing diet last 7 days?

There is no real mystery to this – we have simply discovered that this is the optimum time to fully reboot your system and let those incredible nutrients take effect.

It is long enough to let the vitamins flood through you and have a significant impact, to rid yourself of toxins and refresh your whole being from the inside out. At the same time, 7 days is a short enough time period to be sustainable, practical and enjoyable while being highly effective.

In just 7 days you can lose up to 14lbs, improve the condition of your skin, your digestion, your immunity and turbo-charge your fitness potential.

At the most serious level, it will lower your risk of having a heart attack or stroke. It is a relatively short period of time, but one which can transform your health and leave you glowing with vitality.

Read on and discover how juicing can reap health benefits that you may have thought were beyond you... No such thing, thanks to the incredible liquid power of super-fresh fruit and vegetables.

Discover Scientifically-Proven "Shortcuts" & "Hacks" to Lose Weight FASTER (With Very Little Effort)

For this month only, you can get Linda's best-selling & most popular book absolutely free – *Weight Loss Secrets You NEED to Know.*

Get Your FREE Copy Here:
TopFitnessAdvice.com/Bonus

Discover scientifically-proven tips to help you lose weight faster and easier than ever before. With this book, readers were able to improve their weight loss results and fitness levels. So, it's highly recommended that you get this book, especially while it's free!

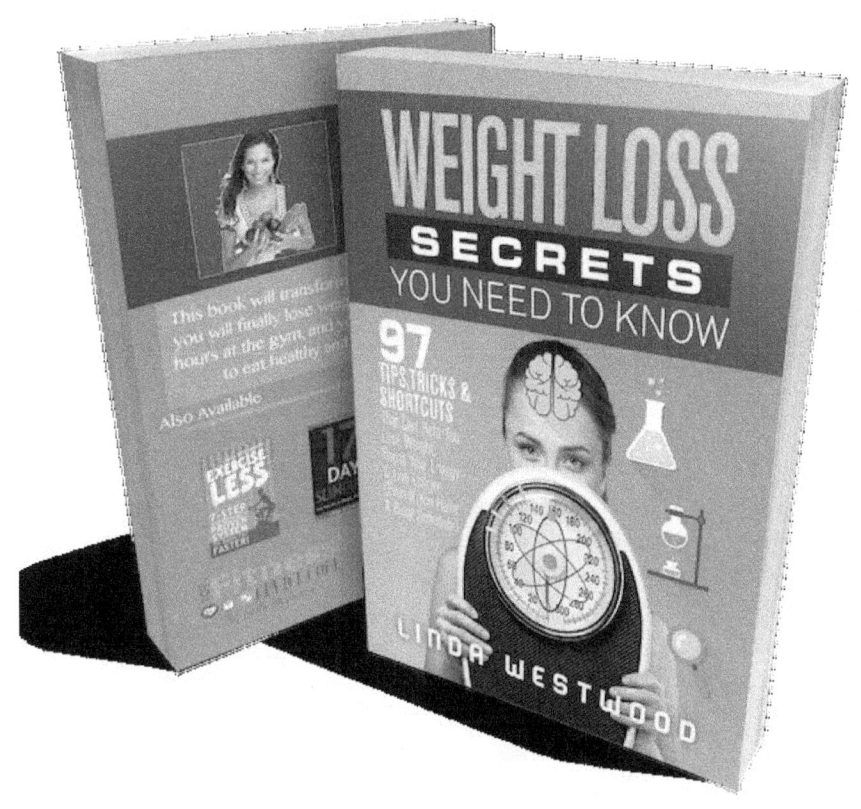

Get Your FREE Copy Here:

TopFitnessAdvice.com/Bonus

Chapter 2

Why Juice to Lose Weight?

So, here's the question – what can juicing *really* do for you? Can it really help you to lose weight?

The short answer is absolutely yes!

When you take the right approach to juicing, the weight really can melt away, for quick and lasting results. If you are new to juicing you may not realize the full, outstanding potential of a true juice diet.

But first things first – how exactly does the juice work such wonders for weight loss?

Why Juicing Leads to Weight Loss

There are a number of reasons why juicing leads to fantastic weight loss. Here are the main weight-busting benefits of this juicing diet:

- Freshly juiced vegetables yield high quantities of nutrients for remarkably few calories. Fruits are also packed with nutrients, although they contain natural sugar so their juice should be drunk in moderation. With an 80/20 veg to fruit juice balance, the calorie total remains low (although you never have to count) and you will have the optimum results for effective weight loss.

- Juicing super-charges your system with the nutrients outlined in Chapter 1. Within days you will find that your system is functioning better than ever and, crucially, your metabolism will be firing on all cylinders, which promotes faster weight loss.

- Freshly squeezed juice is largely made up of water, which is great news, since so are we! The human body is comprised of around 60% water. It is therefore extremely important for good health to remain properly hydrated. Our digestive system and metabolism is fuelled by water, so a liquid diet can really fast-track weight loss.

- Living on juice for 7 days means you are eliminating other dietary baddies that may be causing you to hold extra weight. Out goes any excess starch, sugar, alcohol and fat, in comes deliciously fresh nutrients, water and fiber. Your body will thank you for it by rapidly dropping the pounds.

- Another important point to consider is that 7 days of juicing is simple to do and easy to stick to. With a good juicer and readily accessible vegetables and fruit to pummel into power juice, you can have a relaxing and enjoyable week. Far easier than cooking up complicated and expensive recipes every day, so there's nothing to prevent total success...

- ... which means that when it comes to fast, safe, effective weight loss, juicing is good news all round!

Total Detox Through Juicing

The good news only gets better. Not only does juicing help you lose weight in a very healthy but fast way, it also helps you rid your body of nasty toxins, cleaning your system from the inside out.

The truly great thing about vegetables and fruits is that they are bursting with all kind of goodies that we often overlook in our regular diet.

Detoxing is not just about feeling better from all the things you are not eating and drinking, i.e. caffeine, alcohol, additives and so on, although this is obviously important.

It is also very much about the things you are putting into your body that work brilliantly to cleanse your system.

Here are just a few of the many natural ingredients that detox your system fabulously:

- Lemon juice is well-known as a detoxifying juice, one which gets your metabolism going, so a splash of this is always a good thing - it can also add 'zing' to some of the green juices.

- Strong colors bode well in fruit and veg, especially dark green in vegetables. Kale is full of powerful phytochemicals, while the chlorophyll in spinach is a first-class blood cleanser.

- Spirulina is a type of micro-algae and it is an ultra-healing detoxifying agent, so look out for recipes with a touch of this natural beauty.

- The natural superfood chlorella has detox properties, which help to eliminate mercury and other toxins.

- Beetroot is naturally full of antioxidants, plus nitrates, which allow more oxygen to flow in your blood and can improve performance in exercise.

- Ginger is packed with helpful compounds and has anti-inflammatory and antioxidant properties.

- Pomegranate is a very powerful antioxidant, even more so than green tea.

- Cucumber is superbly alkaline and soothing, so drink as much as you please to give you insides a treat.

This is just a short sample of the many detoxifying fruits, veg and plants you will enjoy on the 7-Day plan. All of the fresh ingredients that you juice will yield a wealth of natural goodies which will support or boost detoxification. PLUS, as they have naturally high-water content, you will continually be flushing your system through with water.

Doesn't Detoxing Have Side Effects?

The short answer is yes, it certainly can have side effects, but this is essentially a good thing as it means the toxins are leaving your body. We are living with more toxins than ever before in our busy, demanding modern lives. Chemicals in and on our food, in our drink, chemicals in skin creams, cosmetics and sprays, chemicals on our clothes... it is a veritable blizzard of toxins.

No wonder we are showing up with more allergies and intolerances – to stay healthy it is more important than ever to regularly detox.

The 7-Day Weight Loss Juice fast will do this brilliantly for you, which is why you may have the odd mild side effect.

When you begin to eat more natural foods that are superior in quality, in other words lots of fresh fruits and vegetables that are packed with nutrients, your body naturally responds to this vastly improved diet.

It sets about getting rid of all the inferior material, waste and tissues in order to make way for the new, superior materials. It then uses the new materials to create brand new, healthier tissues.

Unsurprisingly, with all this positive activity going on inside your body, you may notice changes, especially when it comes to the expulsion of toxins.

For instance, when you cease eating or drinking any stimulants, "fixes" that you may normally have every day like coffee or chocolate, you may experience headaches or migraines. This can be quite a common side effect, since it happens when your body smartly eliminates toxins like caffeine from your tissues and transports them in your bloodstream.

As these toxins travel on their way to their ultimate destination where they will be eliminated, they can cause mild pain or discomfort in the form of an aching joint, or headache and so forth.

You may experience other changes in your body during a detox of any kind. When you start taking in natural food that is of a much higher quality, it triggers the start of a regeneration process in the body.

Part of this process may incorporate a slowing of the heart rate, which you may feel translates as a form of lethargy or inertia.

If this does happen to you, do not worry and do not give up. Just remember that they are the evidence of an exciting internal regeneration process, which on average may take about 7 days up to a couple of weeks, depending on the level of toxicity in your body.

Use this time as a gift - take advantage of it as a period of rest, let your body recuperate and get ready to continue improving its own tissues. You are growing lots of new cells and literally becoming a new person!

Don't be surprised if you feel a little tired. Just remember – it's working!

Have patience and rest assured that experiencing minor ailments is just a temporary state of affairs. Take heart by trying to embrace these inconveniences as proof that your body is changing for the better, moment by moment.

Knowledge is power and forewarned really is fore-armed – now you can relax during your detox knowing that you are not getting ill or going downhill, you are simply regenerating yourself.

In fact, with a few simple, pleasurable additions to your daily routine, you can maximize the effectiveness of your juice detox.

Max Your Juice Detox

If you are going to the effort of planning and carrying out a juice detox, you certainly want to do it as thoroughly as possible, right?

All the more reason to pick up a few more good habits, which will detox you faster and deeper, for more, lasting benefits.

Enjoy a Sauna

As you may be aware, our skin is our largest organ and responsible for the elimination of toxins to a huge extent. Most of us appreciate our skin but we should also learn to love our sweat.

Sweat, or perspiration if you prefer, is an amazing substance when you think about it – it contains scientifically measurable amounts of toxins that have been safely removed from the tissues.

It therefore absolutely makes sense to sweat more, especially when actively trying to detox!

For thousands of years there has existed a basic philosophy of striving to enhance human detoxification.

The Romans had their grand and decorous public baths, the Turkish relished their baths or hammams, the healthy Scandinavian had their saunas, and the Native American tribes had their sweat lodges.

In modern times, saunas can be found in gyms and health clubs, or even private homes.

We know that saunas are good for us because essentially and at a primal level, they *feel* good for us. We can feel the poisonous waste being drawn from our pores and the heat warming our lungs.

Nonetheless, for most people saunas are a very occasional treat. Why don't we spending more solid sweating time?

One reason may be accessibility, but also some people find the high temperatures uncomfortable. They should be aware that there are now more low temperature saunas.

A typical sauna is anywhere from 160 – 180°F. Most people cannot stay in such a small hot room for more than 15 minutes. The less common "thermal chambers" are set to around 100 – 120°F, so you can realistically stay there for much longer and sweat more.

But where you choose to go is not the point, the point is depuration.

Depuration is a fancy name for washing away toxins. The term is also used by fishmongers, when oysters, clams, etc., are rinsed with running water, to swill away toxins. The water essentially carries the toxins away. Our sweat works in the same way.

Enjoy your time when you're in a sauna! Try doing a really good workout before you get in if you want to sweat more. Alternatively, go straight from the office and relax in the heat – the important thing is just to sweat!

Saunas can play a hugely important part of any detox regime. It will only boost your progress, so you have nothing to lose. If you have the time try doing it for 30 minutes daily, as part of your 7-Day Weight Loss Juice fast.

If that is too difficult, doing it once or twice during the week will also make a difference and make you feel good.

Just remember, sweating is extremely good for you. The more you sweat, the more pollutants are drawn out of your skin.

Learn to love depuration. However, make sure you remember to shower thoroughly afterwards, before you simply reabsorb them.

Dry Body Brushing

As the body's largest organ, the skin receives a third of all the blood circulated in the body. It follows that, when the blood is carrying toxins, they will be eliminated through the skin, a major organ of waste elimination.

So, taking care of this organ makes sense if you care about your health.

The benefits of dry skin brushing include:

Increasing the circulation to the skin, which is reported to reduce the appearance of cellulite. Cellulite is not just unsightly in appearance, it is lumpy-looking toxic material which has accumulated in the body's fat cells.

While there are some creams that claim to improve the appearance of cellulite, none of these expensive unguents has been widely proclaimed to be undeniably effective.

Dry body brushing on the other hand is relatively inexpensive – you just need a brush and a little time each day. The brushing helps shed dead skin cells and actively encourage the renewal of new skin cells.

This results in new skin, which looks smoother, brighter and clearer. As an added bonus, dry skin brushing may also help rid the body of annoying ingrown hairs.

However back to the main point – detox.

Dry skin brushing helps to greatly improve vascular blood circulation and lymphatic drainage. It releases toxins and promotes the discharge of metabolic waste. This means that after some dry brushing the body can function more effectively.

The nervous system benefits too as the process of running over the skin with a dry brush stimulates nerve endings in the skin – that's the lovely tingling feeling.

As if that were not enough, the act of dry skin brushing has been found to improve muscle tone and redistribute fat deposits more evenly, getting rid of that 'bumpy' appearance.

Furthermore, dry skin clogs pores and therefore helps your skin to absorb nutrients in a far more efficient manner.

For anyone who is serious some pleasant detox assistance, simply get into a routine of dry brushing every morning before your shower or bath.

It is very easy and you don't need to sign up to some exclusive spa to enjoy this health treat. All you need to do is buy a natural bristle brush (not one made from nylon or synthetic materials). Make sure that it has a long handle, since that way you will be able to reach all areas of the body.

Here's exactly how you do it:

Set some time aside before you plan to have a bath or shower.

Take the brush and work in gentle circular, upward motions, followed by longer, smoother strokes.

When you brush, always begin at your ankles and work in upwards movements towards the heart. There is an excellent reason for this - the lymphatic fluid flows through the body towards the heart, so it's important that you move the brush in the same direction.

The only exception to this rule applies to your back. Brush firmly from the neck down to the lower back.

After your ankles, slowly move up to your calves and knee area, thighs, stomach, back and arms. Don't brush too hard over the softer and more sensitive skin around the chest and breasts, and make sure that you never brush over inflamed or broken skin, sunburn, or skin cancer.

After you have given your body a thorough brushing make sure that you do then have a shower to wash away the dead skin cells and released toxins.

If you would like to invigorate the skin even more and further stimulate your blood circulation, then alternate the temperature of the shower, turning the control from hot to cold as you wish.

After you have showered, do apply a lovely nourishing moisturizer. Keep it unfragranced and natural if you can (otherwise what was the point of the detox?).

Try pure cocoa butter, or coconut oil; argan oil is great for problem areas like scars or stretch marks. Then – your skincare work is done. A little friction, washing, temperature change and hydration can work absolute wonders!

Keep doing it and you could considerably lower your levels of toxicity, which is good for your health in a wide variety of ways.

But if you are going to the trouble of juicing, along with saunas and a bit of dry skin brushing, what exactly is there to gain from a juice detox plan?

The Benefits of a Good Juice Detox

There are many reasons why you will look and feel amazing after detoxing. A proper juice detoxification program is the health gift that just keeps on giving!

With this 7-Day Weight Loss Juice you will:

1. **Enjoy a Great Energy Boost**

    The vast majority of people feel far more energetic after they have been on a really good juice cleanse diet. So many of the less healthy foods that we take in every day clog up and hamper our systems.

    This is an incredibly common modern problem and stopping the flow of sugar, trans fat, saturated fat, caffeine and alcohol and instead filling up with only what our body needs and loves - including lots of that all-important water is - the best thing we can do for ourselves.

Plus, it really is enjoyable to feel zestful and full of energy. Juicing lovers say that it is a wonderful feeling of the most natural, healthy, 'high on life' kind. No wonder more and more people are trying juicing for themselves!

2. Get Rid of Excess Waste

Detox allows the body to release excess waste, which is clearly the primary point of detoxing.

After an effective detox, the liver will be able to work more effectively and with added vigour, as will the kidneys and colon, which means your body will be able to purge itself of harmful toxins.

It is essential to keep the toxin load in your body as low as you can if you want to remain in the best health. High levels of toxins have been associated with all kinds of digestive and other disorders, or even severe illnesses such as cancer. A great juice detox like this one will reboot your toxin-elimination system extremely well.

3. Lose Weight, Naturally

We have looked at why juicing helps with weight loss in a natural, rapid, safe and effective way. However, looking beyond your 7 days of juicing pleasure, you are likely to want to enjoy continued good health. That is why we use the term 'reboot' – it can be a new start and a brilliant way to change old habits.

Make the most of your 7-Day Weight Loss Juice experience by also using all that new-found energy to move around more – walk, dance, work-out and you'll feel fitter than ever and the weight will stay off.

4. Strengthen Your Immune System

With major organs like your liver and kidneys functioning better and with toxins being released, your body is better able to absorb critical nutrients. One of the most important is Vitamin C, which is vital for your immunity. Also, dark green vegetables, ginger, oranges and lemons are among the natural foods which help to cleanse the lymphatic system.

Lymph is a colorless fluid, which contains the immune cells, which protect the body, so it is vital to your health that your lymphatic system functions properly.

5. See Your Skin Glow

As your body's largest organ, your skin is extremely important – it both supports and reflects your condition of health. A vital function of the skin is that it allows us to sweat and this is another way that we get rid of toxins. You may wish to enjoy a sauna as part of your detoxifying regime, in order to sweat out those toxins as much as possible.

As a result of your 7-Day Weight Loss Juice, you are likely to notice your skin looking clearer, smoother and more glowing. Detoxes of this kind can also improve conditions like acne or eczema in some instances.

In fact, detoxifying may cause your skin to itch a little at first, but this will pass. The glow, however, will last for as long as you keep your fruit, veg and water intake at beneficial levels, which includes making them a key part of your daily diet after you stop juicing.

6. Change Your Dietary Ways

We all love a new start now and again. Rebooting your health with a detox can mean the start of a whole new era for the way your body looks and feels. When you do something every day it can become somewhat automatic, even if it is harming your health and happiness. It can be incredibly hard to break those ties to sugar, alcohol, and fried foods and starch overloads.

A juice cleanse gives you permission to start afresh with your diet, in every sense. Rather than just 'give up bad foods', you are gaining delicious, nutritious, new habits that could easily last a lifetime. In fact you will feel so good, you will want them to!

7. Think with a Clear Mind

One of the favorite benefits reported by juicing fans is a much sharper, clearer mind.

This makes sense – think about how your mind feels after you eat a sugary piece of cake or too much pasta.

A sluggish body is never the best way to encourage lively thoughts. On the other hand, spring-cleaning your body will almost certainly encourage your mind to feel brighter too.

The removal of toxins and addition of nutrients really does boost every area of your health. Plus, you should be brilliantly hydrated, which is far better for concentration.

8. Love Your Lustrous Hair

Every cell in our body is affected by our nutrition and that includes our hair. The strand beyond our scalp is effectively dead, as all the growth is in the follicle, so keep it thriving with a detoxing regime. Some people say that after a juice cleanse they can feel the difference in their hair as it becomes softer, shinier and it grows quicker.

Lustrous hair is a good indication of top-to-toe health.

9. Lighten Up

This does not necessarily mean your mood, although that often happens too – it refers to that lovely light feeling that you have on the 7-Day Weight Loss Juice plan.

It makes complete sense – you are ridding your body of excess waste and toxins, your good hydration may have cured any constipation, you are not stuffing your body with heavy foods AND you are losing weight.

Little wonder you feel lighter! The trick is not to panic and misinterpret the feeling as 'empty' or 'hungry' – you will be absorbing everything your body needs to thrive and no more. Enjoy the feeling of no longer being weighed down – the sky's the limit!

10. Look and Feel Younger

Aging is caused by various factors, including the damage done to the body by free radicals. By boosting your intake of antioxidants, you are combatting the process that results in the visible signs of aging, such as wrinkles and coarser skin.

But the anti-aging benefits are not simply cosmetic - you can, of course, very directly affect your lifespan through your diet. We all now know that a diet, which consists of eating large quantities of fried food, is likely to result in a shortened lifespan for most people.

By the same token, a highly nutritious, low toxicity lifestyle that involves some regular physical activity is one that will not only result in you feeling your best, but also living longer.

11. Breathe Fresher

Bad breath can have several causes – but detoxing may really help.

Living without eating spicy, greasy foods, drinking alcohol or coffee (and of course not smoking) is bound to do your breath a real favor. However, there is more to it than that.

If you have bad digestion, or a sluggish colon, it may directly impact on the freshness of your breath.

Get everything moving nicely with a thorough detox and, after a possible couple of days when it may worsen due to toxins being expelled, your breath will noticeably benefit.

12. Feel a Profound Sense of Wellbeing

You should never underestimate the power of detoxing with juice. As well as the countless great things it will do for your body, it is also excellent for the mind and soul.

Many juicing fans report both greater energy and a profound sense of wellbeing, which has a positive impact on all other areas of their home, work and love lives. Feeling incredible – light, bright, hydrated, healthy, regular and perfectly nourished - can lead to great things.

In fact, it can ultimately lead to a far better life in every way... so there is no time to waste – let's get ready to juice!

I hope that you are enjoying this book so far, and if you could spare 30 seconds, I would greatly appreciate you leaving a review on Amazon.com.

Chapter 3

Getting Prepared

Now that you completely understand just how great juicing is for you, it is time to prepare everything you need to the carry out the 7-Day Weight Loss Juice fast.

You do not lead a lot of complicated equipment, just a good juicer, plenty of fresh produce and some simple but highly effective juice recipes. We provide the all recipes for you in this book and we will come to those shortly. But first...

What Makes a Great Juicer?

There are many types and makes of juicers on the market now and if you have never used one before the choice can seem a bit overwhelming. But once you get to know a few basic about what the best juicers can do for you, the choices become much easier.

The main types of juicer are:

Centrifugal

Very popular, they are fast and effective at extracting a lot of juice. Whole fruit and veg can be fed into a tube which has a serrated blade at the bottom, in a bowl that is spinning at 12000 rpm.

This creates the centrifugal force which separates the juice from the pulp, so that pure juice comes out of the tap.

- **Pros** – Fast, simple to use and clean, no pre-slicing of fruit or veg required, many are at affordable prices.

- **Cons** - Not as much juice as masticating models, can be loud to use, juice does not stay fresh for as long due to the heat and air.

Masticating

These types of juicers pulverize the fruit and veg, which you feed into it via a tube. They vary: there are those that can take whole fruits, those which are slower and deliver great juice, those which can juice wheatgrass and those which feature twin gears and are the strongest and often the most expensive juicers.

- **Pros** – High quality juice, quiet.

- **Cons** – Slower than a centrifugal juicer, more expensive on the whole.

Fusion

This is a new type of juicing technology, which combines masticating and centrifugal techniques, giving it the 'fusion' name.

- **Pros** – High quality juice, quiet, affordable.

- **Cons** – Slower than centrifugal models, some peeling required, no wheatgrass juicing.

Once you have considered what your juicing priorities are, including the types of fruit and vegetables that you mostly want to juice and how easy any model is to clean (dishwasher safe is great), you will be closer to knowing the best model for you.

Before you buy, here are a few final do's and do not's:

- Don't simply be tempted to go for the most expensive model on the market – go for one tailored to your needs, you may save money.

- Don't, on the other hand, be tempted to choose something so cheap it will barely last the 7 days – think of buying a juicer as investing in your own health.

- Do read consumer reviews on the latest models to get the inside story on using each juicer.

- Don't think that a blender or anything other than a purpose-built juicer will do the trick. You need a proper juicer that you can rely on – especially when you will be drinking several juices a day and nothing else.

- Do look out for special offers and package deals that include juice bottles for when you need to store juice and drink juice on the go.

- Do go for a juicer that you really like using, even if it is that bit more pricey – that way, you are even more like to keep juicing in future.

Once you have met and purchased the juicer of your dreams, you just have to give it plenty of fresh fruit and vegetables to get busy with – even more fun!

Nature's Fuel – Fruit and Vegetables

Buying the fruit and vegetables to put in your juicer will be some of the best shopping you ever did in your life.

What could be more fun than selecting food that creates fuel to make you feel better than ever? Totally guilt-free food shopping with a weight-loss pay-off - fantastic!

So, what type of vegetables are the best? Some, like beetroot and kale, have already been mentioned for their antioxidant properties.

There are many, many more to choose from. We have put many of them into one big shopping list, but urge you not to buy every single one in one go.

Why? Nutrient degradation – the loss of nutrients in fresh food after it has been harvested.

Unless you are getting all your fruit and vegetables straight from the tree (big garden!), you will have to plan to buy the produce that has been on the shelf for the shortest time.

The ideal would be to buy just what you need for each day and the next morning's breakfast juice and to get your fruit and veg as fresh as possible.

This would also leave you free to pick your favorite recipes as you please – they are so good you may wish to repeat some.

However, we appreciate that everyone has pressing demands on their time like work, children and so on, while others live miles from the shops and may not be able to devote the requisite hours for hunting down organic produce on a daily basis.

So, to make life easier, we have provided a list of all the fruit and vegetables that are used in all of the 7-Day Weight Loss Juice fast recipes.

You can look up the recipes that take your fancy and mark off those ingredients on this list.

However, you want to do it, it is just a handy tool to make your juicing flow more smoothly. You will find the Shopping List at the end of this chapter. But back to our fruit and vegetable selection.

Many people wonder 'does organic produce make any difference?' The short answer is 'absolutely, yes!' Organic fruit and vegetables have been grown without the use of any artificial substances, chemical fertilizers or pesticides at all.

The growers abide by strict guidelines to ensure that the produce is unadulterated. The result is that organic fruit and veg has been found to be higher in antioxidant compounds and far lower, even of negligible levels when it comes to in toxins, metals and pesticides.

This is obviously extremely important when you are aiming to detoxify your body. Choose organic. There has been plenty of debate around the world as to whether organic food is worth the bigger price tag.

It may not be possible for everyone to buy it every day at current prices, but when it comes to something as special and important for your health as a juice cleanse, it is worth trying to make the stretch.

Besides, you can always grow your own!

Not yet convinced? Don't believe us, here are some facts and figures taken straight from the Soil Association:

Production methods really do affect quality

Extensive analysis has proven that the quality of food – including fruit and vegetables - is influenced by the way it is produced. Chemically sprayed produce has consistently been found to be of a lower quality than the best organic produce.

Fresh organic food contains even more antioxidants

Organic crops - most essentially, in this case, fruit and vegetables, but also cereals - have significantly higher concentrations of antioxidants and/or polyphenolics when compared with their non-organic equivalents.

This includes more antioxidant, anti-inflammatory, cancer prevention, cell protecting compounds including phenolics (19% higher), flavanones (69% higher), stilbenes (28% higher), flavones (26% higher), flavonols (50% higher).

If a consumer were to switch to eating only organic fruit and vegetables, this would entail a 20-40% increase in antioxidant and/or polyphenolics consumption. An essential point to note that this increase in these miraculous natural compounds comes without a downside as there is no corresponding increase in calorie intake.

Fewer pesticides

Pesticides residue can be found on non-organic crops. The occurrence of pesticide residues is in fact four times higher on crops that have not been grown organically.

Non-organic fruit has the highest pesticide frequency (75%), compared to non-organic vegetables (32%). In stark contrast, pesticide residues were only found in 10% of organic crop samples.

Less cadmium

Cadmium is a toxic heavy metal, one that is carcinogenic to humans. The analysis detected 48% lower concentrations of cadmium in organic crops.

Less nitrogen

Nitrogen concentrations – which have been linked in some studies to an increased risk of certain cancers such as stomach cancer – were discovered to be significantly lower in organic crops. So again, buy, or harvest, organic produce.

Yes, organic fruit and vegetables are certainly more expensive than your average chemically-farmed crop. They may even look more knobby, weird or misshapen. But they are fruit and vegetables of the highest nutritional value, so don't compromise on this point unless you really have no choice.

Besides, organic is no longer niche. It is easier than it has been for years to find fresh organic produce and remember, the fewer the food miles, the less nutrient degradation may have occurred.

Go to farmer's markets and seek out your local organic specialists. Have fun, ask questions, and try rare varieties of old favorites, like apples.

Shop around if you have the time and if you are spoilt for choice, broadly aim to buy the organic produce that has most recently been in the ground or on the tree – it is a fun, healthy challenge!

What Juices Do I Drink?

The beauty of the 7-Day Weight Loss Juice is that we provide all the recipes for you – you will find them at the back of this book. Make these juices to replace three 'normal' meals each day and solid snacks.

There are recipes that you can enjoy for breakfast, lunch and dinner, even as snacks, and they are all tasty and interesting. We outlined before that the best ratio of fruits to vegetables for a juice fast is 80/20.

Therefore, while there are plenty of sweeter juices, which many people like for their breakfast, the other meals are largely comprised of vegetable-based juice. There are exceptions and some 'green' juices, packing a punch of kale perhaps, which may also contain an apple, some lemon, avocado pear or another fruit.

Don't think in terms of conventional recipes - it is all about loading up your system with super-nutritious juice that also tastes great. The recipes in this book are designed to be fun to make, with accessible ingredients, but critically each one is bursting with fresh nutrients and should be drunk as soon as possible.

Once you get into the swing of juicing and you start to feel the effects, you may be amazed at how excited you get about making your next delicious fresh juice!

Think Juicy, Think Health

You may be all revved up and raring to go already, or you may be finding it hard to adjust to the juicing mindset and feel anxious about getting started.

Here are a few thoughts to put your mind in the right place before you start juicing. Remember, this is an exceptionally healthy, all-natural way to lose weight – no gimmicks, nothing to worry about!

You have flexibility, so if you would rather replace one vegetable for one you prefer, you can, although ideally for one with similar nutrients (you can refer to the list in Chapter 1 which will help).

Stay focused and upbeat as you do your juice fast – it is important to make sure you are determined to finish it.

You may have moments when you think 'why bother?' or 'I need solids, now!' – this is totally natural. At those times just think of the weight that is slipping off your body and maybe even re-read the benefits of a detox outlined previously.

Think of it as the most wonderful health treat you can give your body!

Most of all, relax and prepare to love your juice cleanse. It really is that simple and effective.

Next, we take a look at exactly how to do it for the best results. But first of all, here's that helpful Shopping List.

Naturally, no quantities are stated because that is up to you and the recipes that you choose. Don't forget, it really is best not to buy everything all at once for freshness' sake and because there is simply so much in the list.

Read the recipes, find your favorites, choose what produce you need and then buy it when you need it, as fresh as possible. Simple!

Shopping List

- Alfalfa
- Apple
- Asparagus
- Avocado
- Basil
- Beetroot
- Blueberries
- Broccoli
- Blood orange
- Bok Choy
- Brussels sprouts
- Cabbage (green)
- Carrots
- Cauliflower
- Celery
- Chili
- Coconut water
- Coriander
- Courgette
- Cranberries
- Cucumber
- Dandelion greens
- Fennel (plus fronds)
- Garlic
- Ginger
- Green grapes
- Jalapeno
- Kale

- Lemon
- Lime
- Mango
- Mint
- Oranges
- Papaya
- Parsnip
- Parsley
- Pear
- Pineapple
- Pomegranate
- Radishes
- Red grapes
- Red bell pepper
- Red cabbage
- Rocket
- Romaine lettuce
- Ruby grapefruit
- Savoy cabbage
- Spinach
- Spirulina (powdered)
- Strawberries
- Swiss chard
- Tomatoes
- Turnip leaves
- Watercress
- Watermelon
- Wheatgrass (powdered)

Chapter 4

How to Do the 7-Day Weight Loss Juice

This chapter takes you step-by-step through the best, most effective way to carry out the 7-Day Weight Loss Juice fast.

However, this is not a rigid plan and as you read on you will discover that there is plenty of built-in flexibility to make sure that you get a brilliant 7-Day Weigh Loss Juice plan that is totally tailored to you.

10 Tips for Following the Plan

The plan is extremely easy to follow and allows you a fair degree of freedom at the same time as offering lots of no-brainer health ideas to choose from.

Here are the basics:

1. Start your day by waking up your system. You may well be thirsty and while our breakfast juices are refreshing, they are intensely nutritious.

    We recommend that you drink a glass of still water with a slice of lemon in it to cleanse your system soon after you wake up. You may wish to make it warm water, especially if you normally drink coffee or tea – it is a super-healthy alternative.

2. Next, choose any of the delicious breakfast recipes from Chapter 8. There is a real variety in the selection that we are suggesting, which means two things.

   Firstly, it means that you will never be bored as each juice is different from the last.

   Secondly, and essentially, you will be able to choose from a range of juices that, between them, offer a vast array of nutrients – great news!

3. Once you have enjoyed your breakfast juice, ideally you will indulge in some form of activity to maximize the benefits of all that wonderful natural energy.

   We all need to work, but perhaps you might walk or cycle to the office, or jog around the park before you start work for the day. If you don't have time, even just taking the steps all day rather than using the lift or escalators will be beneficial.

   This is not compulsory, as the 7-Day Weight Loss Juice plan will certainly work without exercise, but this will make it even more effective by revving up your metabolism as well as boosting your mood and morale thanks to all those incredible endorphins and of course burning calories faster.

   Moving more is your friend and a great companion to the detoxifying, cleansing, and weight-busting juice diet.

4. When you are ready, select your lunch from the juices in Chapter 9. These are, on the whole, more savory and substantial, as any good lunch should be. Simply choose the flavor combination you fancy from the wide variety of recipes.

   As regular juicers, we would advise you on one point, do not take lunch too early in the day, especially in the first couple of days when you may feel a bit hungrier. The trick is to wait until you have a real appetite for your juice – it may not be strictly at 1.00pm, it could be at 2.00pm, or 4.00pm.

   However, do not wait until you are absolutely ravenous or you may 'over-drink' or even be tempted to break your juice fast - your stomach will tell you when it's time.

5. If you feel a dip in energy in the afternoon, do not sit and suffer – feel free to enjoy a delectable, entirely nutritious snack juice. There are a bunch of them to choose from and you will find them in Chapter 11!

   Think of them as natural sweets or little power-bombs of flavor. Choose just one per day and enjoy guilt-free snacking at last!

6. Post-snack, you should be feeling good – energized, nourished and full of vitality.

   Once again, consider this as an opportunity to enjoy some fresh air and a bit of exercise. Walk the dog, go to the gym, take the kids to play in the park, or even just walk enthusiastically around town picking up the freshest fruit and veg you can find for your next day's juices.

7. When it is dinnertime, try to balance your choice of juice with whatever else you have drunk that day.

   For example, you may love carrots, but don't select a heavily carrot-based juice for breakfast, lunch, dinner and your snack. Mix it up and you will reap huge benefits in terms of nutritional variety and health benefits, not to mention the boost in terms of morale – no one wants to be on a boring and bland diet.

   Also, try not to consume too late in the evening. This is also a good rule for when you return to solid food. You do not want to pump any calories into your system just before you go to sleep as they are more likely to be converted into your fat stores and sit on your belly or hips rather than nourish you.

   There is far less chance of that with these low-calorie, super-healthy juices, but what is a realistic potential problem is that the sheer energy boost you receive from these stimulating, nutrient-packed juices may keep you awake if drunk too late in the evening!

   Don't drink any after 8pm and perhaps do a few stretching exercises to wind down before bed.

8. If you think that some of the juices will not be exactly to your taste, don't be afraid to substitute one natural ingredient for another one.

    For example, if you can't stand spinach, replace it with watercress, or Savoy cabbage, for example.

    Try to replace like with like in nutritional terms as closely as you can – i.e. don't swap kale for a banana and be careful not to overload on sweetness during the day even though they are all-natural sugars.

    That said, it is ESSENTIAL that you feel free to choose at will – it is your body, your favorite natural juices, your own 7-Day Weight Loss Juice plan!

9. Small but important prep note for when you are getting ready to juice your fruits and vegetables.

    If in doubt do NOT peel your fruit or vegetables. The highest concentration of nutrients often lies just beneath the skin, or even in the skin itself so you really don't want to miss out on all that natural goodness.

    If you have bought organic produce, then there is absolutely no reason to peel everything, as the skin will not be covered in pesticides. Only peel your produce when the skin is thick, pithy and/or bitter, as with grapefruits and other citrus fruits, pineapples, kiwi fruit and so on.

The likes of carrots, apples, cucumber etc. certainly do not need to be peeled and, in fact, you will be detracting from their nutritional content if you do peel them. Put the knife away!

10. One final note. Drink ONLY your chosen juices, do not eat solid foods, and do not drink coffee, tea or alcohol of course, for the duration of this 7-Day plan.

    Apart from one exception - the fantastic news is that in addition to the juices of your choice you can drink as much life-giving water as you like.

    Water, plus intense fruit and vegetable goodness – for the next 7 days, that really is all that your body needs.

In fact, we positively encourage a lot of water as well as juice – read on to learn more about this and other tips for success.

Once again, thank you for reading this book, and I hope you're getting a lot of valuable information. I would greatly appreciate it if you could take 30 seconds to leave me a review for this book on Amazon.com.

Chapter 5

Top Tips for Success

As with any weight loss plan, if you remember a few key points and adopt the right attitude, then you will certainly succeed in dropping the pounds.

You are already on the right track and have proven that you have the desire to do the fast by reading this much of the 7-Day Weight Loss Juice plan. Now all you have to do is bear in mind some important considerations that will keep you motivated and determined to succeed.

We have made it all as easy for you as possible, but we still understand that even just 7 days can feel like a long time unless you totally embrace and enjoy the juice fast.

Read through our excellent top tips. They will guide, support and encourage you as you go through what could be the healthiest, most beneficial, nutritionally most rewarding 7 days of your life.

Drink Water

That means lots of it.

Start the day with water, end the day with water; drink lots of water all day long. This has numerous benefits.

It will flush out nasty toxins more effectively and keep you superbly hydrated. It will keep your metabolism and digestion firing on all cylinders. It will, critically, fill you up, quench your thirst and finally it will make sure that your delicious juices remain special, as proper meals and are not just gulped down to quench your thirst.

The benefits of water are immeasurable. Want to know exactly why?

Benefits of Water

Good old H2O is terrifically important, but frightening amounts of people who are lucky enough to have easy access to clean, free-flowing supplies do not drink it in sufficient quantities.

Or we load it up with sugar and chemicals and say it is 'improved'.

Don't believe the hype. Water always was and always will be the best drink on earth.

In case you need reminding, here are a few scientific reasons why:

1. **Keeping Body Fluids Balanced for Optimum Health**

    The human body is made up of around 60% water. It is a fundamental part of us and without enough it vital functions start to falter – from digestion to the maintenance of body temperature.

As we are constantly losing water through perspiration, respiration and excretion, we must top up our water levels regularly.

So, stay hydrated and, following your 7-Day Weight Loss Juice fast, beware of coffee and alcohol's dehydrating effect on the body.

2. Proven to Help Control Calorie Intake

Whilst water isn't a magic potion (although it must surely be the closest thing to one), whenever you make the choice to drink it instead of a sugary, fatty or alcoholic beverage, you are making a choice that will help you with weight loss.

Also, when you eat food or drink juices that contain lots of water they will fill you up much more.

3. Supports Muscles for Exercise

Muscles tire without enough water. When exercising, it is vital to drink fluids regularly – around 17 ounces before, and plenty during and after. A well-hydrated body is more efficient; it will burn energy better and repair muscles following exercise more effectively too.

4. Keeps Skin Glowing

Healthy skin needs plenty of water to keep the layers hydrated and looking good.

Drinking more will prevent avoidable dryness and some wrinkles, so if you spend money on moisturizers don't forget the most important hydrating fluid of all.

5. Supports Kidney Function

Kidneys need generous amounts of water to help them in their vital role of excretion – and too little can result in kidney stones.

Our cell's waste products include blood, urea and nitrogen, which the kidneys turn into urine to be passed out of the body.

You can easily tell whether you are properly hydrated as your urine should be somewhat colorless and without odor. If not, drink more water.

6. Supports Bowel Function

If you drink enough water, you reduce the chances of experiencing constipation. A properly hydrated body enables the gastrointestinal tract to work at its best, especially when plenty of fiber is consumed as well.

Simply drink plenty of water all day long on your juice fast, especially between your juice meals.

If you work in an office, always keep a bottle of water on your desk.

If you're at home, you should constantly have a glass on the go – aim to drink 6-8 large glasses each day.

Now, back to the other tips for success…

Try Not to Obsess About Food

If you just live for food and can't wait for your next gourmet thrill, you'll have trouble sticking to any fast plan.

Good food and great company is some of life's wonderful moments. But remember – you will be consuming intense hits of the best foods that the planet has to offer while on this fast!

Try to change your mindset and really get behind what you are eating. If you find that tough, all you have to do is read through the list of nutrients once again and you can get carried away on a tide of enthusiasm for all the great things that you are doing for your body.

Don't Eat by the Clock

This is a very common mistake people make, mainly because our jobs and lives dictate a certain amount of routine. It may seem practical to eat at the same time every day without fail, but if left unchecked it becomes a negative life habit.

After all, it makes no real sense, unless you also eat exactly the same things every day – in reality some days you are likely to feel hungry earlier or later than others.

It therefore makes no sense to pre-arrange food. Wait until you need it!

Enjoy Your Food Shopping

You will be buying a lot of fruit and vegetables for this 7-Day Weight Loss Juice plan, so do it in such a way that means you really enjoy it.

If can find a great organic produce supplier near to you, don't hold back, get to know them. It may be more expensive than your usual grocery shopping, but it really will be worth it.

If the organic store is an independent one and you let them know that you will buy large quantities all week, you might even be able to secure a cheeky discount!

Don't Starve Yourself

On this fast, you really will not need to skip any juice meals or go without nourishment when you need it. All of the plan is low-calorie and has been balanced so that if you stick to it, you will lose weight.

However, if you start missing juice meals, the chances are that you will simply end up really hungry and either end up grabbing the nearest solid, fatty snack, or, if you carry on, you will slow down your metabolism and find the weight even harder to shift than before.

So, relax and drink your low-calorie, high-nutrient juice.

Tell Your Friends

In order to feel totally comfortable and confident about your fast, you need to be able to share the exciting news about the plan with your nearest.

Tell them in straight terms that you are doing the 7-Day Weight Loss Juice fast and that you will not be eating solid for a week.

Make sure that they understand that you will be packing yourself full of highly nutritious vitamins and minerals; delicious and totally natural juices for 7 days. Once they understand that you are not starving yourself, they are bound to offer you their support.

But what does that support mean, in practice?

It means not waving biscuits and slices of chocolate cake under your nose; not minding if you rain-check on coming over to dinner for a few days; understanding if you are full of chat about how energetic and amazing you feel – that's what friends are for!

Avoid Eating Out (It's Just For 7 Days)

Unless you know an amazing organic juice bar near you, you had better cancel any restaurant invitations for a few days.

If that's impossible, they may not mind you quietly sipping your juice in a corner, across the table from your partner who is eating steak, but why put yourself in that uncomfortable position?

Rearrange your diary a little and give yourself full license to stay at home and juice just as you please.

Do a Before and After Selfie

Motivate yourself by taking a photograph of yourself at the start of your juice cleanse, when you may be looking and feeling and bit overweight, pasty and blurred around the edges.

Then, simply look forward to taking another photo after 7 days of drinking pure, fresh juices and water.

You may be amazed at the difference in your appearance – normally a slimmed down profile and an incredible glow.

Aim for those 'Skinny Jeans'

Motivation is vital when losing weight.

Find a fabulous piece of clothing that you are longing to be able to get into and use it as your inspiration.

It might be a lovely, new cocktail dress in a smaller size, or your favorite jeans from 5 years ago. Hang it up, take it out, look at it, and keep trying it on.

If you love it, keep on track and you'll soon be wearing it!

Get Your Beauty Sleep – Essential!

A University of Michigan study shows that getting one extra hour's sleep per night could help a person drop 14 pounds in one year.

When you are sleeping, it is true that you're not eating, but also lack of sleep has been proven that people become hungrier and more prone to reaching for sugary, fatty, high-calorie snacks.

Don't break your fast because you are over-tired.

If you have trouble getting to sleep, then try doing some yoga before bed, or soaking in a hot bath. Sleep well, recharge your batteries and then face the day full of energy.

Think it makes no difference?

Here are some essential facts about why regularly getting a bad night's sleep can make you fat:

- A faulty sleep pattern, meaning either too much or too little, we play a role in obesity and causes inflammation within the body.

    Inflammation may participate in the poor functioning of hormones and is the enemy of those who are trying to stay healthy and lose weight.

- A study in Sleep magazine tracked adults' belly fat over five years. People who slept five hours or less, or eight or more hours, per night gained more belly fat than those who slept between six and seven hours per night.

- In another study, just one poor night of sleep of about 4 hours was enough to significantly affect the effectiveness of insulin in the body.

   This means the body cannot metabolize carbohydrates and fats properly, which will make a weight problem worse.

- In fact, in one study, reducing the subject's sleep time from 8 hours to 6½ hours caused their metabolism of fat of to fall by two-thirds.

- Ever noticed how after a bad night's sleep you seem more prone to eat sugary or carbohydrate-loaded foods like bread, cakes, cereals and pasta?

   This is due in part to the fact that lack of sleep causes raised levels of the "hungry" hormone ghrelin.

- Also, it lowers levels of the hormone leptin, which tells you when you are full. Not great for when you are trying not to overeat.

- More bad hormone news when you don't get your beauty sleep. You may suffer from increased levels of the stress hormone cortisol. Excess cortisol in your system can cause the body to lay down more belly fat.

- Yet another study showed that preventing men from sleeping for just one night led to them eating significantly more the following day.

- As if all that were not bad enough, one final study showed that when we have slept badly, if we going food shopping the next day we buy higher calorie items than when we sleep well.

Celebrate Each Victory

Reward yourself as the pounds drop off to keep you motivated.

Of course, you must not fall back on old habits though and crack open a vat of wine and order in a few pizzas – but celebrate in a way that does not sabotage your 7-Day Weight Loss Juice fast – with a beauty treat like a massage or facial, a new pair of shoes (which you can enjoy even as you shed further pounds), or some jewelry.

Tell people about your success and be proud of yourself!

Plus Another VITAL Tip - Get Moving!

You probably already know this (and may have been simply ignoring it), but consider it to be a final, essential 'bonus tip'.

Exercise to burn far more calories and speed up your metabolism.

For example, if you play an hour of strenuous tennis, swimming or doing weights in the gym, you'll burn around 600-700 calories.

That's approximately equivalent to one cup of sugar. If you exercise regularly and are also eating much less in caloric terms, you will certainly lose weight.

Want to stave off those irritating cravings?

Make sure you exercise. We have been shown in studies to reduce our food intake by as much as half when we take exercise.

Do at least 30 minutes exercise each day and reap enormous benefits not just for slimming but for your wider health and happiness.

Whatever you choose, make it something you love and try and make it a habit. It does not have to be long-distance running or hardcore reps at the gym.

How about any of these ultra-fun options?

- Adult gymnastics
- Aqua aerobics
- Beginner's kick-boxing
- Bikram yoga
- Beach volleyball
- Capoeira
- Flamenco
- Hiking through amazing scenery

- Hula hooping
- Ice skating
- Jazz dancing
- Just Dance computer game
- Karate
- Nordic Walking
- Obstacle courses
- Off-road mountain biking
- Rock climbing
- Rollerblading
- Rowing somewhere scenic
- Salsa
- Skiing
- Skipping
- Spinning to top tunes
- Tae Kwon Do
- Tap-dancing
- Tango
- Trampolining
- Ultimate Frisbee
- Urban dance
- Water polo
- Wii Tennis, Wii Fit etc.
- Zumba

Any of these fun options will do, or if you want some competitive fun, why not take up a team sport like hockey, football or netball?

Choose one, choose ten, mix it all up, and shake it all about. Just flood your body with endorphins, feel great and lose weight.

Chapter 6

Continue Losing Weight After the Juice

We have no doubts that this is an exceptionally effective 7-Day Weight Loss Juice Plan, but what about life after the juice?

You are about to discover a way forward that ensures you will lose further weight if you wish and keep the weight off.

The Morning After

So, let's say you have just woken up after the 7th night of your juice fast. You did not cheat, you slept and exercised well, you drank water and you enjoyed the experience – firstly, congratulations! You did it!

But what next? What happens on Day 8? The short answer is – whatever you want.

You could go back to old ways of eating, but the chances are that they are what got you to the point of needing to the point of needing to lose weight in the first place.

Happily, most people will be feeling so good that the last thing the feel like doing is reaching for a cheeseburger and fatty fries. They will want to carry on feeling fantastic and maybe also losing weight.

The great news is that you certainly can carry on, with a few simple modifications that will help you enjoy a sustainable and more long-term healthy diet.

Straight Back to Solids?

The short answer is 'not necessarily'.

On day 8, you have earned a break from juice, so mark the occasion with a little light protein and some vegetables for your breakfast.

We would recommend a poached egg on a bed of watercress and tomato, if that takes your fancy. Alternatively tuck into some fresh fruit, tomatoes on spelt toast, or even a simple plate of crunchy crudités made from your remaining vegetables.

Post-Juice Plan

You may wish to ease into your post-juice phase by alternating solid meals with juices. This really is an excellent approach, particularly if you wish to lose further weight, or even to simply embark confidently on a healthy new lifestyle. You don't want to launch yourself into a frenzy of calorie counting and you do not need to either.

This is a sample plan that you may wish to either adopt or adapt after you finish fasting, according to your own tastes. Throughout the days following your juice fast, make sure you keep on drinking plenty of WATER.

Others who are considering purchasing this book would love to know what you think. If you could spare a few seconds, they would greatly appreciate reading an honest review from you. Simply visit the page on Amazon.com.

Day 1 Post-Juice

Wake-up

Drink warm filtered water with a slice of lemon, or hot water if you prefer. Make this a lasting habit, perhaps replacing your over-stimulating caffeine-bomb of coffee. It's both soothing and cleansing.

Breakfast

1 medium poached organic egg, a large handful of fresh watercress, and 1 medium ripe tomato, cut into wedges.

Get moving

Walk the dog, cycle or walk to work, do some gardening, go to aqua aerobics at your local pool, take the stairs on the underground, etc.

Mid-morning snack (optional)

A small handful of mixed seeds

Lunch

Now's the time to give your digestion a rest and reassure it with a fabulous fresh treat. Opt for a delicious juice from our list, such as Alfalfa Forest or BroccoBeet Booster.

Get moving AGAIN

You will be feeling absolutely great so make good use of it with a little light exercise (or lots of vigorous exercise if you prefer!).

Afternoon snack (optional)

Try something light and soothing like a Cucumber Calmer to help your digestion re-adjust to solids. It is simple and delicious, perfect for the first day post-juice.

Dinner

Now it is the time to try a little warm food, as the chances are you will be feeling like a change after a week of cold juice. But as this is a watershed, don't go back to charring everything to a crisp, thereby ruining the nutritional content entirely.

Instead, enjoy suppers that have being lightly cooked with little fat or starch, like this stir-fry:

- Water chestnuts
- Baby sweetcorn
- Red and green peppers
- Bean sprouts
- Carrots

Lightly 'fry' in an inch of searing-hot water for just a minute or two until the beansprouts and water chestnuts are just turning translucent.

Heat can destroy certain nutrients to an alarming extent.

For example, cooking removes about two-thirds of the vitamin C in fresh spinach. Therefore, you don't want to overcook your stir-fry and kill the fantastic nutrients contained within these fresh foods – just warm them through and keep them as close to raw as you possibly can.

Day 2 Post-Juice

Wake-up

Enjoy a refreshing, hydrating, cleansing glass of warm water or hot water with that lemon!

Breakfast

Juice time!

Choose a tasty, zingy option to kick-start your busy day, such as Kale Super-Booster or Get Up and GoGo Juice.

Get moving

If you have to go to work in an office, try to incorporate a walk – park further away or get off the bus a few stops earlier and walk through town.

Mid-morning snack

A satsuma or kiwi fruit for a juicy hit of Vitamin C.

Lunch

Enjoy some crunch in the form of a superfood salad. The fiber will fill you up and the high-water content will keep you hydrated.

Try something along the lines of this for a good balance of vitamins, minerals and more:

- Rocket
- Watercress
- Spinach
- Pomegranate seeds
- Spring onion
- Tomatoes
- Cucumber
- Avocado
- Red chili
- Mushrooms
- A sprinkling of mixed seeds

AND

If you are feeling in the mood, add just a few freshly seared king prawns for some irresistible lean protein – you've earned it!

Afternoon snack

You may not feel like one after such a satisfying lunch and you will not actually need a solid snack.

But if you do feel like snacking later, try a glass of unsweetened almond milk, which is non-dairy and very low in calories, but full of antioxidant Vitamin E and other nutrients.

Get moving

Try going for a walk with friends, or even colleagues, after work.

Walk home from the office or go for a bike ride to unwind rather than pouring a glass of wine.

Dinner

Keep it light and warm tonight. Try this chicken and mushroom broth:

- 1 chicken breast
- 1 pint or organic chicken stock
- Half an onion, sliced
- A carrot, sliced
- A handful of mixed variety mushrooms
- A handful of flat-leaf parsley

Grill the chicken and cut into bite-sized pieces.

Splash a little of the stock into a saucepan and use it instead of oil to sauté the onions and mushrooms.

When they have softened, throw the chicken pieces into the pan, add the stock and carrot and simmer gently for a few minutes until the carrot is tender.

Serve with the chopped parsley scattered over the broth.

Day 3 Post-Juice

Wake up

Drink some warm water with a slice of fresh lemon.

Breakfast

Grilled tomatoes on spelt toast.

Get moving

Pick a fun activity from the list earlier and try it out.

Rollerblading in the park? Or rock-climbing? The choice is yours, time permitting. If you will be at work, go for a few purposeful walks around the building rather than filling up on coffee and biscuits.

Mid-morning snack

Crunch on a Granny Smith apple.

Lunch

Choose a lovely juice that will power you through your afternoon with energy.

How about a juice such as Hero's Cabbage or Dark Secret Detox?

Mid-afternoon

Crunch on some chunks of chilled cucumber

Get moving

Do something that means you have to either jump around a bit, or cover some distance. Walk or cycle home from work, even jut partway if it is a serious distance.

For example, if you drive to and from the train station 5 minutes away, try going without the car today – it might become a habit.

Dinner

Go for another delicious mix of warm and cold ingredients, temperatures, textures and most importantly nutrients in this salmon niçoise salad.

- Fillet of salmon, grilled, broken into pieces
- 1 Cos lettuce, torn up
- 1 boiled egg, yolk just set
- 8 cherry tomatoes, halved
- Handful of green beans, blanched
- 3 new potatoes, boiled, halved
- A brief drizzle of olive oil

This dinner covers a lot of nutritional bases and it tastes great. Plus, after your juicy week, it will be time to enjoy some oily fish, which delivers some all-important Omega-3 fatty acids (alongside potassium, selenium, Vitamin B12 and more).

Moving Forward

The post-juice phase is important and should not be ignored. The gradual introduction of solid food, alternated with more delicious fresh juice will work wonders for ensuring the pounds continue to melt away.

The trick is not to think 'it's finally over' and tuck into piles of red meat, cheese, pasta and so on.

Also, think twice before re-introducing regular alcohol into your diet, if this is something that you used to enjoy before your juice cleanse.

Alcohol is extremely high in calories. One 175 ml glass of red or white wine contains around 120 calories, champagne contains around 130 calories and a 12-ounce serving of beer contains around 150 calories.

Alcohol essentially has 7 calories per gram versus sugar, which has 4 calories per gram. Think about this next time you are wondering whether to have a glass of wine after work – you will be drinking something more calorific than an equivalent sugar solution.

Amazing, and not in a good way!

So, how do you avoid that back-to-before trap, which may be tempting however much you also love fruit and vegetables?

The most important thing is to listen to and look at your body.

Is it now lighter, with brighter eyes and skin and shinier hair?

Is your digestive system working far more smoothly?

Are you energized and alert, with none of the huge energy highs and lows of the sort that come during and after a session of eating cakes?

If you can answer yes to some or all of the above – and if you properly follow the 7-Day Weight Loss Juice plan you will be able to – then you will be feeling terrific.

Why jeopardize that after such a health-boosting week?

There is no need to put all those benefits to waste, just follow the post-juice phase advice and then introduce other types of protein, including the occasional piece of lean red meat if you wish, plus whole grains, seeds, pulses and healthy fats like olive oil and coconut oil.

Before you realize it, you will already have embarked on a whole new healthy way of life.

Enjoying this book?

Check out my other best sellers!

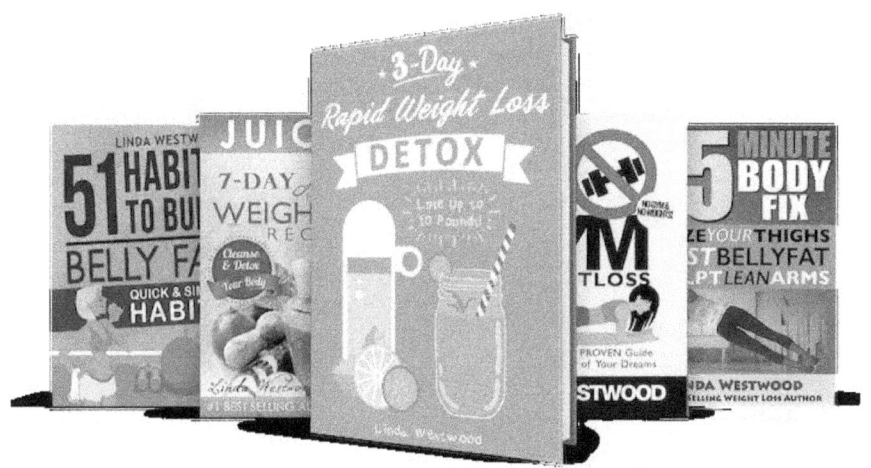

Get your next book on sale here:

TopFitnessAdvice.com/go/books

Chapter 7

Weight Loss Boosting Secrets

Once you have got a taste for juice, you are likely to find it hard to put down. This is great news!

We can often pick up so many bad habits throughout our lives – smoking, drinking too much alcohol, getting hooked on chocolates and much worse – that it makes a literally refreshing change to pick up a very good one.

Now you have discovered the magic of a really great juicing fast, you may want to 'go the extra mile' by carrying out longer juice fasts from time to time. Again, great news!

Your body will love you for charging it up with generous doses of natural nutrients and reward you with better health and further weight loss.

However, you and your body may find a longer fast to be a slightly different challenge.

With the right preparation, however, juice fasting for 14 or even 28 days can be an ultimately enjoyable experience.

Benefits of a Longer Juice Fast

- The best part of doing a further fast that is longer than 7 days, apart from drinking all the lovely juices, is that you will lose more weight.

- Extended second fasts are beneficial for the body because it gives it the uninterrupted time during which real cleansing and healing can take place.

- According to some scientific studies, certain diseases like Type 2 diabetes can even be reversed after a successful long fast.

- Release even more toxins from your cells, which will be eliminated from your body as waste.

- The greatest amount of deep healing begins to take place after around 21 days of an extended juice fast when the cells begin to regenerate using the excellent new nutrients that they are receiving.

Preparing for a Longer Juice Fast

Pick a Date

Choose carefully when you are deciding when to start your 14+ day juice fast. After all it would not be ideal to start it at a time when you know you will be unusually busy, or when you have lots of social occasions that revolve around food booked into your diary.

Go for a quieter stretch of time and work out for how many days exactly you want to carry out your juice fast. At least 3 days to 1 week prior to starting your longer juice fast, you need to prepare your body for the change in eating habits that is about to come.

If you are tempted to have a few quick 'last suppers' consisting of pepperoni pizzas, chips and ice cream before you are due to begin, think again.

This is no time for you to forget why you are doing this – it is not an empty challenge or a stretch of time to be completed and forgotten about – your health is your greatest asset.

So, instead of the hasty burger feasts pre-fasting, do the exact opposite. Cut down on the foods that you might normally eat, including wheat and starchy carbohydrates – bread, baked goods, pasta, rice, potatoes etc.

You should also start eliminating, or at least minimizing, dairy products, eggs and sugar. Reduce the amount of processed foods you eat, cut out artificial soft drinks, as well alcohol. You really do not want to give your body a bigger toxic load to deal with than you have to, so keep the cork in the bottle. As for smoking, if you do it definitely stop that too (ideally forever)!

But it is not all virtue and denial. It's a straight swap of bad habits for good habits, that's all. So, you don't need to go hungry before a juice fast – that would be absurd. You can still eat lean protein like fish, seafood, chicken, turkey and eggs. Just fill up more than usual on fresh fruit and vegetables... plus lots of water.

Get Into Gear

Prepare yourself mentally and emotionally as well. If you would like your longer juice fast to be as successful for you as the 7-Day Weight Loss Juice fast was, then you need to prepare your reserves of discipline and determination.

These are both essential, even if you adore drinking fresh juice – there are likely to be temptations and distractions during a fast of two weeks or more.

Remind yourself of why you are doing the juice program and remember that you now not only know benefits of your juice fast, you have seen and felt them for yourself already. Let this reassure you and make preparing to fast much easier.

Immediately before your fast, start stocking up on organic fruit and vegetables. Make sure you have jars or bottles in which to store excess juice. Have your juicer on standby, clean and ready to go.

You're all set!

Chapter 8

Breakfast Juice Recipes

Breakfast - the most important meal of the day, so the saying goes.

We agree that a good breakfast is essential, so we have devised the most delicious juices we can find to start up your engine in the morning, put a smile on your face and have you dancing out the door. You need a good breakfast to fire up your metabolism for the day. More than any other meal, it is essential for weight loss.

Studies have shown direct links between people who skip breakfast and problematic weight. Conversely eating breakfast boosts a dieter's chances of success.

Regular breakfast eaters have been found to be far more likely to exercise regularly. Plus, people who eat breakfast regularly tend to eat fewer calories overall during the day.

The good news is that you do not have to think twice about enjoying your breakfast with these super-nutritious treats! You will find some sweet and some savory recipes in this chapter, all offering a load of outstanding nutrients.

Even after your 7-Day Weight Loss Juice, you may well wish to continue to keep having a green or fruity juice for breakfast. Millions already do and benefit from the best possible start to the day. Happy juicing!

Get Up and GoGo Juice

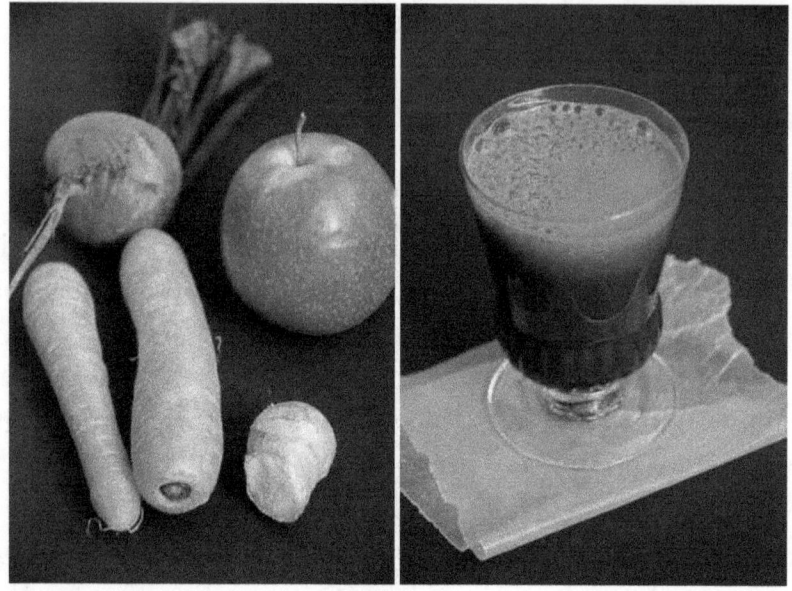

Citrus and root vegetables combine to deliver a tantalizingly sweet and sour, deliciously invigorating juice that delivers lots of Vitamin C, cleanses your liver, blood and digestive system, peps you up brilliantly and prepares you for a busy day.

- 1 large lemon
- 1 lime
- 2 beetroots
- 2 carrots
- 2 apples
- A thumb-sized piece of ginger

TIP – Putting in whole lemon will give a zestier taste, which can verge on bitter depending on the variety of lemon.

If you opt to leave your lemons intact, make sure they are always unwaxed whenever you use them unpeeled – no one wants tiny bits wax bobbing about in their lovely fresh juice!

Green and Gorgeous

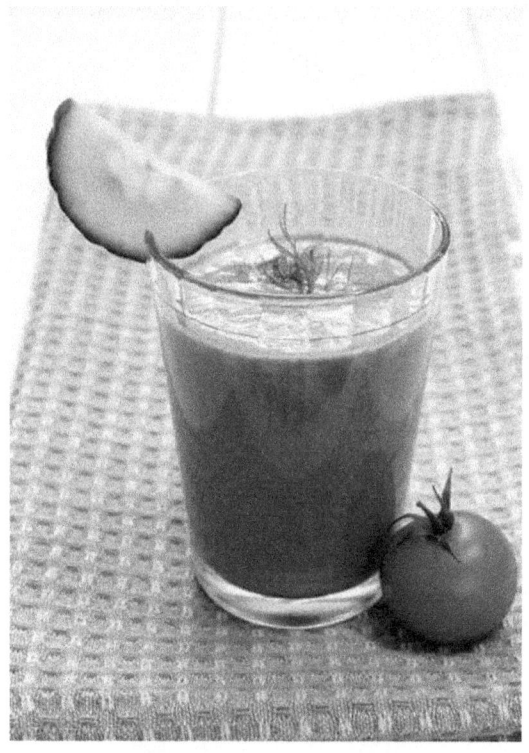

This juice brilliantly balances green fruit and vegetables, plus it adds a few other goodies.

It is a great fresh drink that offers up ingredients with a wealth of antioxidant, cancer-preventing, hydrating, cholesterol-lowering, bone-bolstering, skin-brightening properties... We could go on but you're probably dying to try it!

- 2 apples
- 3 carrots
- 1 medium cucumber
- 10-12 green grapes

- 1 green bell pepper
- 2 large handfuls of spinach
- 1 large tomato

TIP – Add a teaspoon of spirulina and one of chlorella for a super-cleansing boost. Available from good health food shops.

Mango Mamma

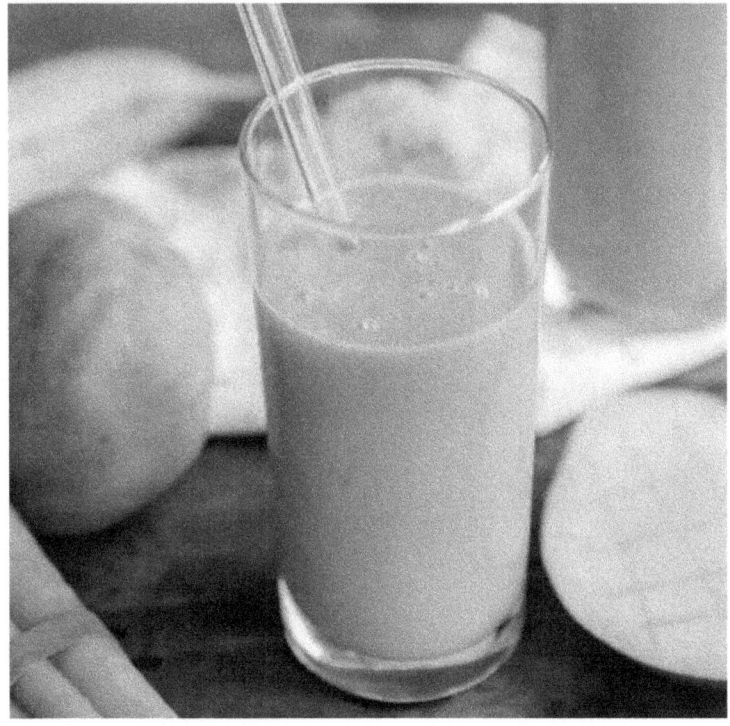

There is something about the taste of fresh mango that signifies a real treat.

The same applies here, which is great news since mangoes are full of C, vitamin A, folate, vitamin B6 vitamin K and potassium.

- 1/4 mango
- 1 blood orange
- 3 strawberries
- 1 large carrot
- 1 cucumber

- A handful of spinach
- 3 romaine lettuce leaves

TIP – Tasty though mango is, don't be tempted to put a whole one into the blend as that might overbalance the sugar levels (and therefore the calories).

Kale Super-Booster

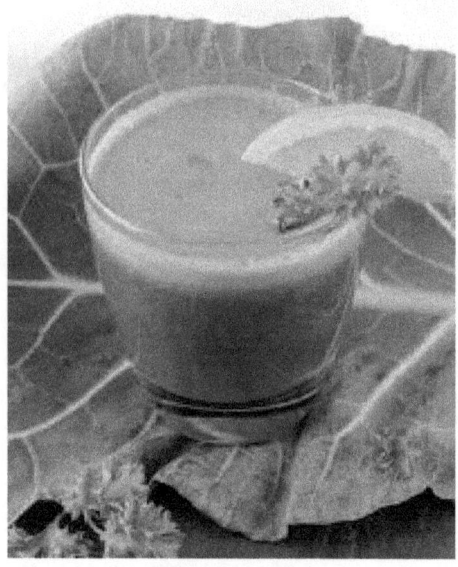

This juice features plenty of kale, the big green giant of detox juicing. Kale is full of calcium, antioxidants and super-healthy, purifying compounds, so drink up!

- 5 large leaves kale, torn in into manageable pieces
- 1 lemon without the zest and pith
- 1 large apple
- A thumb-sized piece of ginger
- 1 sprig of mint

TIP – The distinctive flavors in this green juice makes it perfect for when you want a juice breakfast of substance.

Red Sky

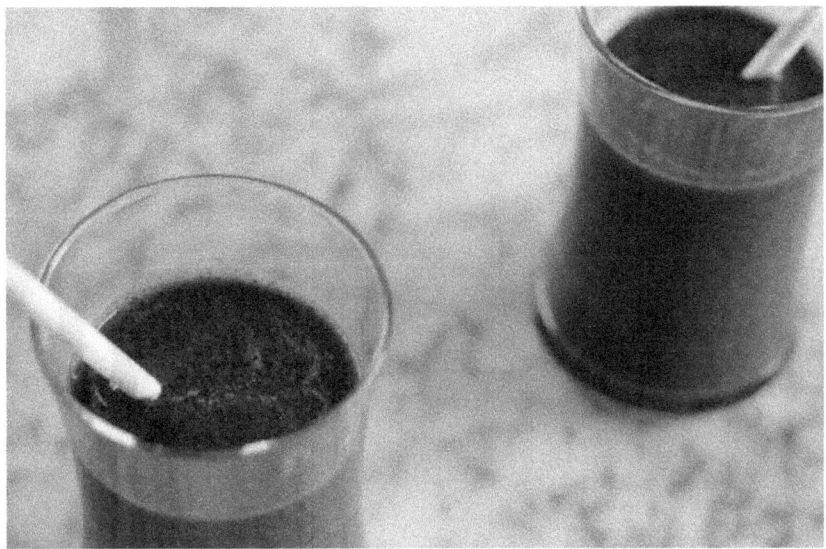

This deliciously sweet, powerfully ruby juice is a complete treat for anyone who wants to fill up on antioxidant superfoods while feeling a little bit indulgent. A gorgeous rich red, it will leave you glowing.

- 1 handful of red grapes
- 1 handful of pomegranate seeds
- 1 handful of blueberries
- 2 apples
- Ice

TIP – 'Red sky in the morning, shepherd's warning' goes the saying. Our only warning with this fabulous juice is to try not to enjoy it more than once during a 7-Day fast as too much of the natural, energy-giving sugars may slow weight loss.

Sweet Charity

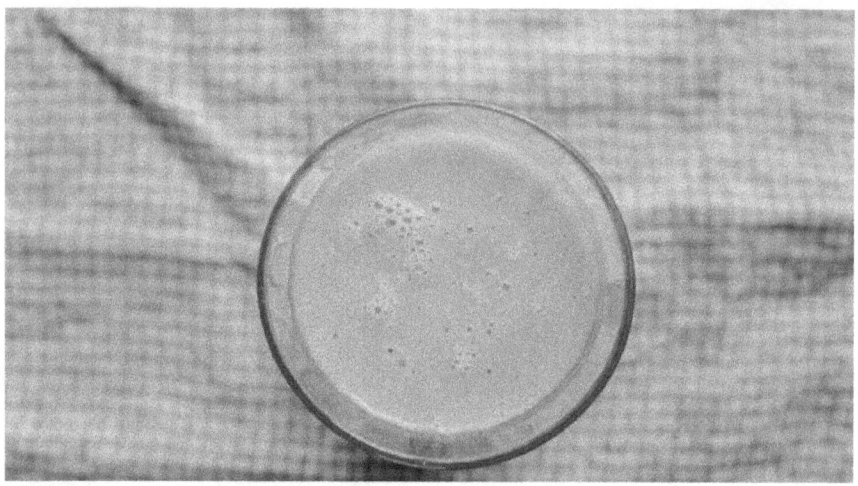

Gently sweet, with a touch of creamy avocado, this juice will soothe and recharge you.

- 1 cup of fresh organic coconut water
- ½ avocado, pitted
- 2 celery stalks
- 1 large handful of strawberries
- 1 beetroot
- 1 lemon, zest and pith removed ice
- 1 apple

TIP – If you love this juice, but want to keep things interesting, make it for another breakfast with different varieties of apple, lime instead of lemon and may throw in a little milk thistle powder if you want to take care of your liver even more.

Jamaica Juice

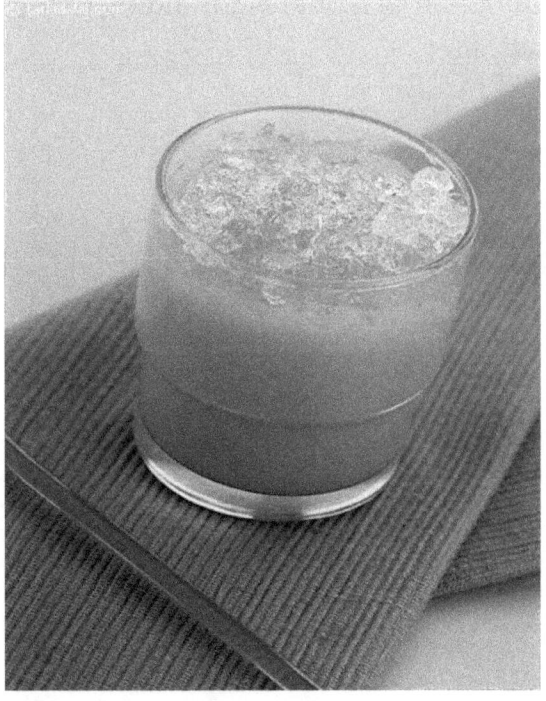

The touch of papaya in this uplifting, flavor-packed, green juice gives it the tropical name. Eating papaya can reduce the risk of heart disease, diabetes and cancer, so tuck in.

- ½ pear
- ½ papaya
- ½ Granny Smith apple
- ½ cucumber
- 1 large handful spinach
- 2 celery stalks
- 1 handful parsley
- 1 small piece ginger

TIP – Makes a lot of juice so fill up once and store some for later. Want it even more tropical? Swap the apple for a large slice of pineapple – it is fabulous for aiding digestive problems and inflammation.

Ready Steady Go

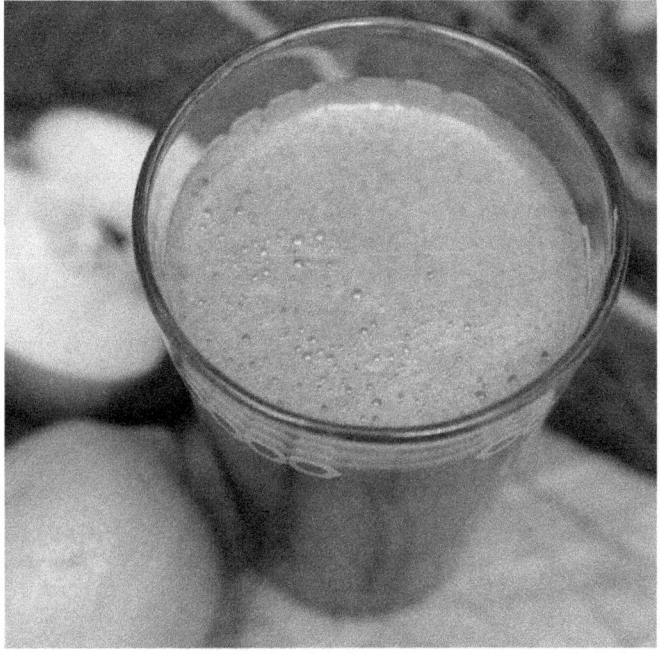

A simple, delicious, effective juice that will load you up with fresh Vitamin C and kick-start your digestive system. A great way to start the day.

- 4 Swiss chard leaves
- 1 green pepper
- 2 apples
- 1 cucumber
- ½ lemon
- 1 piece of ginger

TIP – The younger leaves of the green leafy veg will be less bitter but still highly nutrient-charged.

Ginger Love

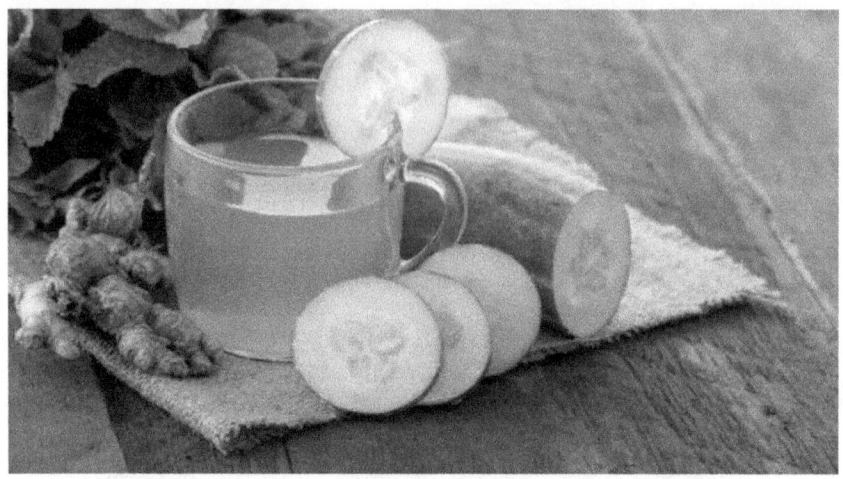

Ginger is our friend. It soothes and stimulates, providing excellent gastrointestinal support – yet another one of nature's wonders. Enjoy this over ice for a great warming-refreshing taste contrast.

- 2 stalks of fennel
- 1 ½ thumb-sized pieces of ginger
- ½ cucumber
- ½ green apple
- 1 handful of mint

TIP – If you love lightly aniseed flavor of fennel, feel free to add more. Fennel has been proven to reduce inflammation and to help prevent cancer.

Sweet Parsnip Skinglow

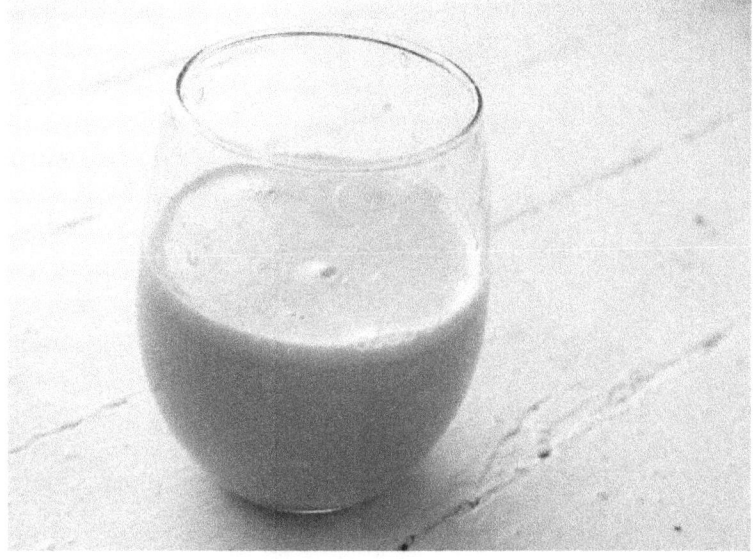

Parsnips taste fantastic, but they are also packed with folate, potassium and vitamin C. The cucumber and green pepper boost skin, hair and nails too.

- 2 parsnips
- 3 carrots
- 1 cucumber
- ½ lemon
- ¼ green bell pepper

TIP – Add a touch of spice if you fancy a warming treat. Cinnamon lowers cholesterol and reduces inflammation so add a good teaspoonful – especially nice in winter! Or it you want to rev up your metabolism and like it hot, try it with a touch of fresh chili.

Super Sunrise

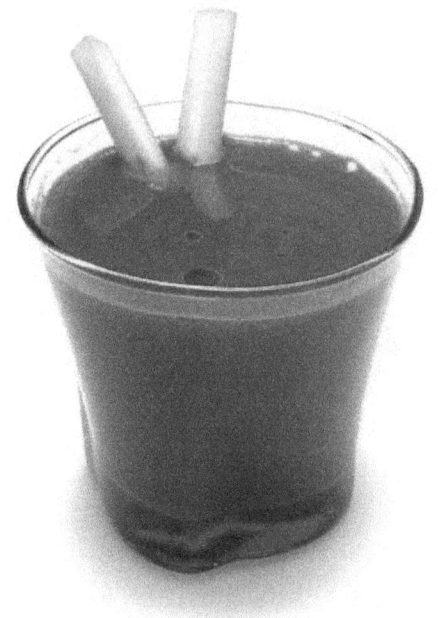

Wake up! Time to enjoy a delicious fruity blend of beetroot, orange and mint. The natural energy and performance-boosting beetroot will be especially great if you about to workout or go for a run.

- 1 medium beetroot
- 2 blood oranges
- 1 large celery stalk
- 5 mint leaves

TIP – If you can pick your mint fresh from your herb garden, so much the better for this natural stimulant. It will also soothe your stomach and give you sparkling breath!

Carrot Caramba

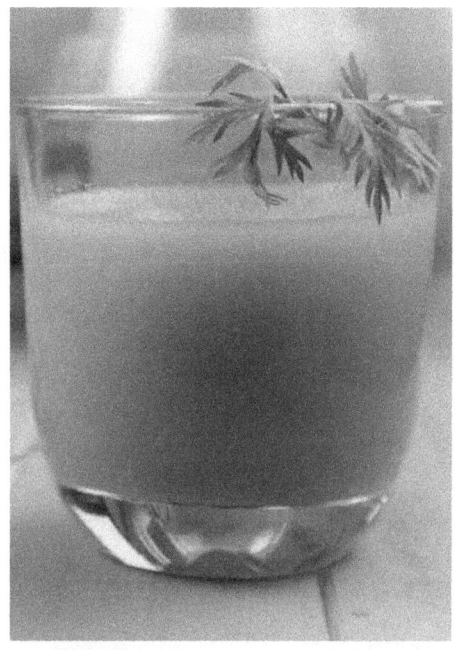

Carrot are a bright orange delight, bursting with natural goodness. They are a one-stop health shop - reducing cholesterol, detoxifying, preventing heart attacks and cancer, improving vision and skin, and reducing the signs of aging, plus much more. Anyone for seconds?

- 2 large carrots
- 1 juicy pear
- 1 thumb-sized piece of ginger
- 1 cup parsley

TIP – If you are feeling a bit light on fiber, very finely grate some extra carrot into your juice, for a tasty fiber top-up.

Tropicaltastic

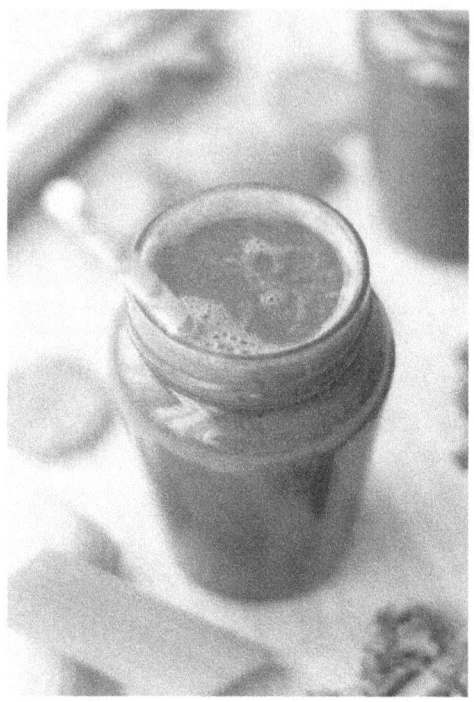

What could be better than a burst of fresh, sweet pineapple and luxurious avocado pear in the morning? Set yourself up for the day in style.

- 2 apples
- A handful of spinach leaves
- ½ pineapple
- ¼ avocado
- ¼ cucumber
- Celery stick
- ½ lime
- Few ice cubes

TIP – This juice is rich in potassium, vitamin C and iron, this boosts immune system, so drink up it you're feeling under the weather, it's a Caribbean break in a glass.

I hope you have learned something from this book so far and would greatly appreciate it if you could leave an honest review on Amazon.com.

130

Chapter 9

Lunch Juice Recipes

Whatever else your day brings, it is important to be able to look forward to a great lunch.

On this juicing fast we have carefully selected more substantial, interesting and savory blends for you to enjoy.

Whether you are at home, at work or on the go, these tasty liquid treats will fill you up and keep you going at the same time as nourishing and cleansing you.

Superleaf Lunch

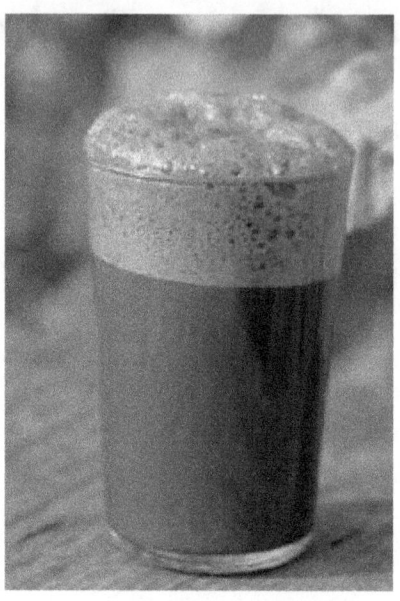

This dark-green, delicious blend packs a real vitamin and antioxidant punch. There is so much good stuff in here it is hard to list it all, but here are the headlines – iron-packed anti-cancer spinach and dandelions greens, also loaded with calcium, peppery vitamin and superfood watercress, ultra-nutritious kale and much more... all with far too many benefits too list!

- 1 handful of spinach
- 3 stalks of celery
- 1 small bunch of dandelion greens
- 1 small bunch of watercress leaves
- 3 leaves of green kale
- 2 juicy soft pears, like Williams variety
- ½ cucumber, peeled

- ¼ lemon
- 1 small handful of parsley

TIP – When you are hungry, go for this great juice. A strong but pleasant flavor makes it like a chilled green soup. Add more watercress if you love a peppery kick.

Carroty Cleanse

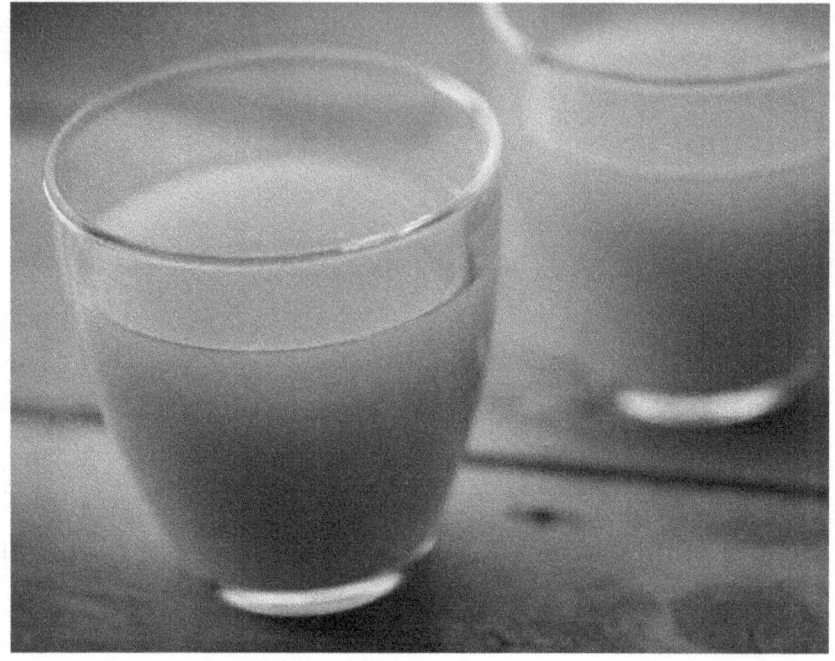

Carrots for antioxidant cancer-fighter beta-carotene and cleansing your liver, spirulina for power-boosting your immune system.

- 6 carrots
- 2 tsp spirulina
- ½ lime
- A handful of mint

TIP - Try this at least once during your cleanse, as the spirulina is a unique superfood which also lowers cholesterol and normalizes blood pressure.

Alfalfa Forest

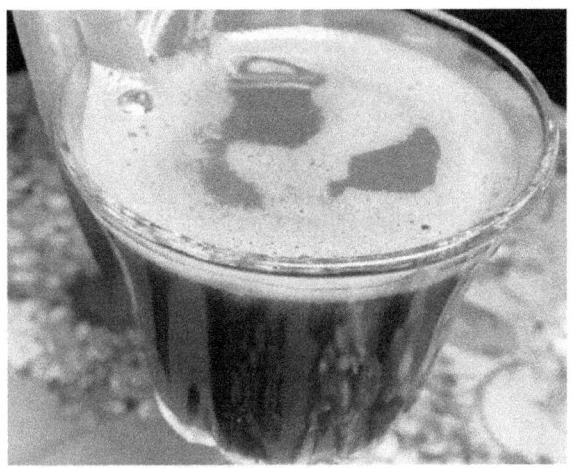

Alfalfa is a delicious sprout, very high in protein, calcium and other minerals, plus B vitamins, vitamin C, vitamin D, vitamin E, and vitamin K. What a star!

- A large handful of alfalfa sprouts
- A handful of kale
- A handful of watercress
- 4 broccoli florets
- 2 apples
- 1 orange
- 1 tsp wheatgrass powder
- Ice cubes

TIP – Always rinse alfalfa sprouts thoroughly before use. Also, don't skip the wheatgrass, it is a protein-rich superfood which contains all minerals known to man, and vitamins A, B, C, E, l and K, plus 17 amino acids. Enjoy!

BroccoBeet Booster

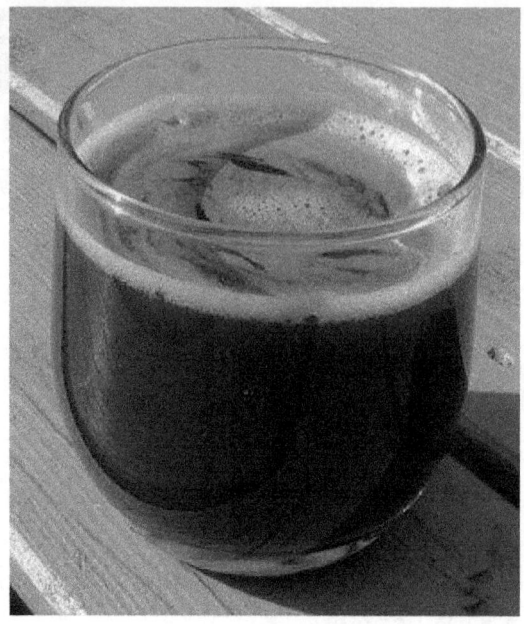

This is a hugely nourishing juice which will amply feed your detoxing body with all manner of natural treats. Ideal when you want a more complex and interesting juice to stave off hunger.

Whet your appetite by recalling that in tests broccoli was proven to prevent the development of cancer tumors by 60 percent and to reduce tumor size by 75 percent! Then you add nitrate-rich beetroot, which lowers blood pressure, plus kale, alfalfa... If this is not a superfood juice, what is?

- 6 florets of broccoli
- 1 broccoli stem
- 2 beetroot
- 2 apples

- A handful of kale
- A handful of alfalfa
- 1 small carrot
- 1 stick of celery
- ¼ cucumber
- ¼ courgette
- A thumb-sized piece of ginger

TIP – Feeling peckish? Further boost your juice with a pinch of fresh, anti-inflammatory chili, to create the best chilled vegetable chili soup you will ever drink!

Cucumber Calmer

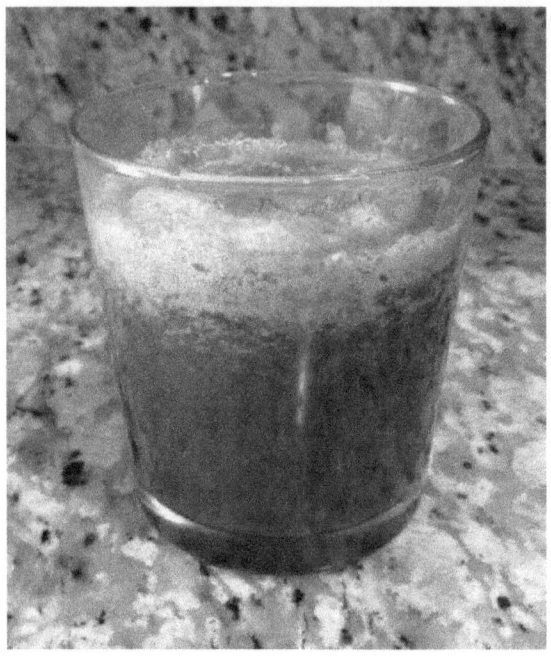

Busy day? Don't get hot and bothered; calm your spirits with this wonderfully light and soothing concoction, which is excellent for the digestion and the blood. The very high water content will refresh you too.

- 2 cucumbers
- 1 handful of spinach
- 1 handful of parsley
- 1 celery stalk
- ½ lemon, peeled

TIP - Don't be tempted to peel your cucumbers, instead reap the full benefits of their vitamin K content.

Hot Gossip

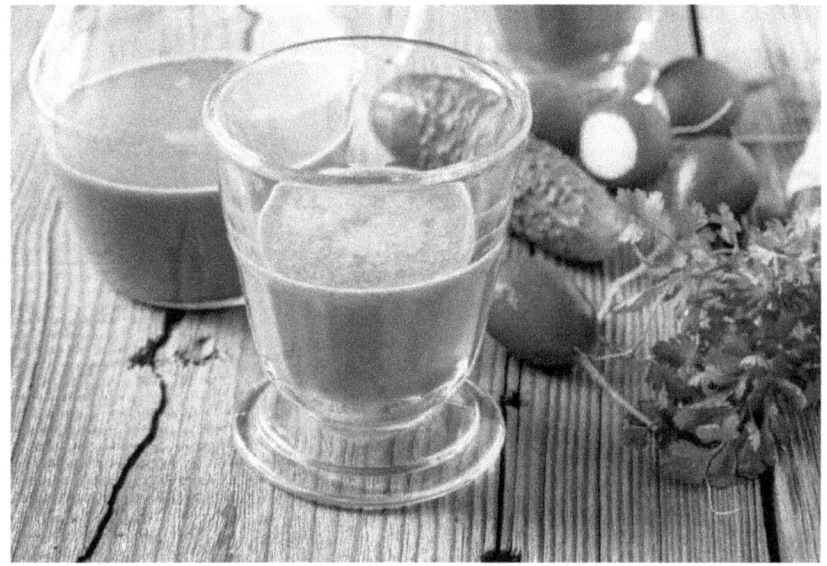

This is a deliciously different detox juice, one that boasts many health benefits. The radishes offer their peppery taste whilst delivering a load of great nutrition. They are excellent for the liver and stomach, acting as a powerful detoxifier and they are fantastic for purifying the blood and eliminating toxins and waste from the body.

The rocket only goes to add to the hot flavour in terms of taste. Meanwhile, it ups the nutrient ante by providing a whole host of them, including folate, which makes it perfect for pregnant women.

- A handful of radishes
- 1 cucumber
- A large handful of rocket

TIP – Think this will be too spicy for your palate? Simply halve the amount of rocket and add in some mild-tasting romaine lettuce. Otherwise, leave it just as it is and enjoy the pleasant sensation of your engine being revved up for the rest of the day.

Feisty Fiesta

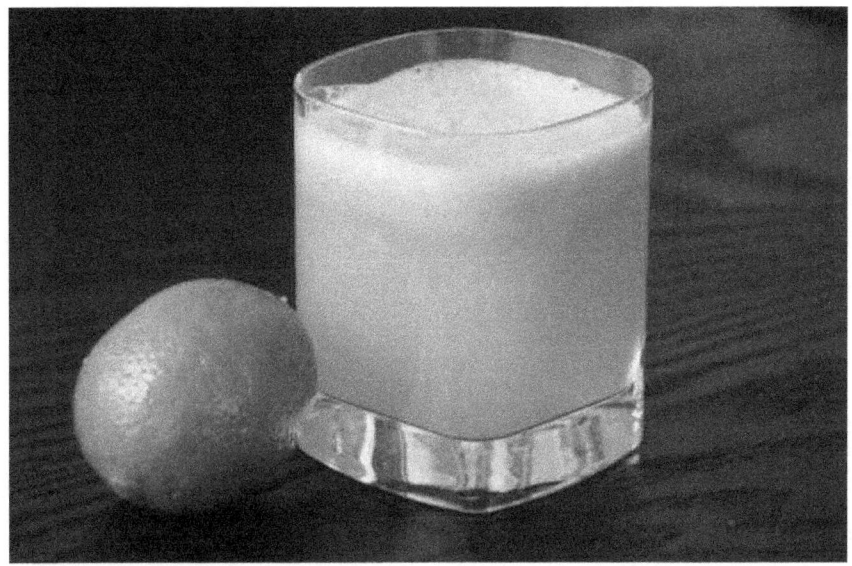

Like a bit of a kick with your fruity juice? You will love this Mexican-inspired treat. The touch of jalapeno will support your metabolism and add spice to the other tasty flavours.

- 1 large pineapple
- 1 Granny Smith apple
- 1 lime
- 1 jalapeno
- 1 small handful of coriander

TIP – If you find jalapenos too mild for your taste, try a little touch of a more fiery number, like Bird's Eye chilli, for example, which will care for your heart and give you a spicy flavor hit.

Hero's Cabbage

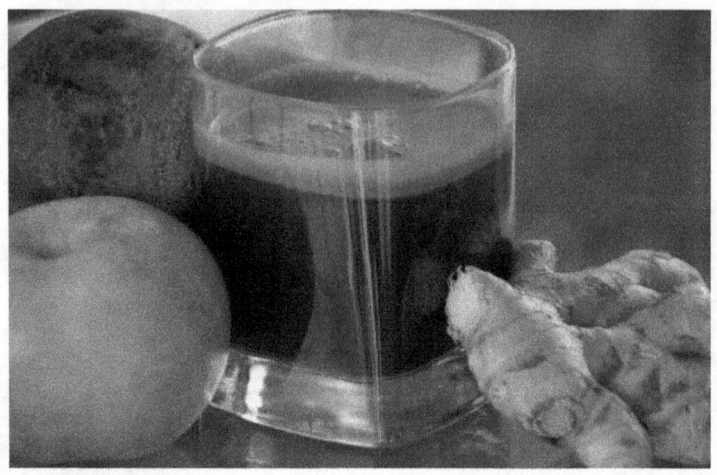

Cabbage is a real treat. It is often taken for granted as 'boring' but it is a superb natural source of sinigrin that converts to AITC, which helps prevent all kinds of cancer. In terms of taste, the red cabbage is sweeter and more peppery, so add more if that's your preference.

- 1/4 Savoy cabbage
- 1/84 red cabbage
- 2 celery stalks
- ½ beetroot
- 1 Granny Smiths apple
- 1 large carrot
- 1 lemon, peeled
- 1 thumb-sized piece of ginger

TIP – If you can get your celery stalks whole, i.e. with leaves, this is best, for added phenolic antioxidant.

Pepper Punch

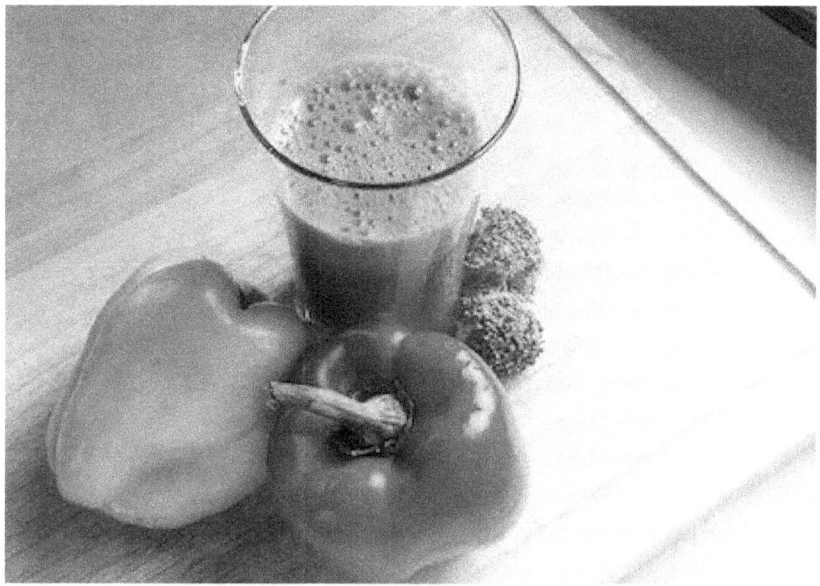

Fancy something zingy yet filling for lunch? Red salad peppers are bursting with beta-carotene, vitamin C, folate, numerous B vitamins, vitamin E, vitamin K, iron, manganese... and plenty of delicious flavor.

- 2 large red bell peppers
- 1 small cucumber
- 6 florets of broccoli
- 1 carrot
- 2 celery stalks
- 1 whole lime
- 1 handful of fresh basil

TIP – If you fancy, blend in some small slices of chilli.

Dark Secret Detox

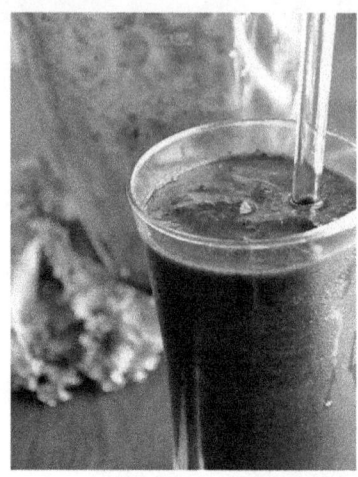

This wonderful juice is dark in color and overflowing with natural goodness. It contains lots of detox favorites, plus the lightly aniseed fennel tops, with their unique phytonutrients and Vitamin C, add an unusual touch (perhaps that's the 'secret').

- ½ green cabbage
- 4 celery stalks
- 4 carrots
- 1 beetroot, untrimmed
- 1 whole lemon
- A handful of coriander
- A small handful of fennel fronds
- A thumb-sized piece of ginger

TIP – Don't overdo the fennel fronds unless you want a strong taste of licorice – less is more.

The Mild Quencher

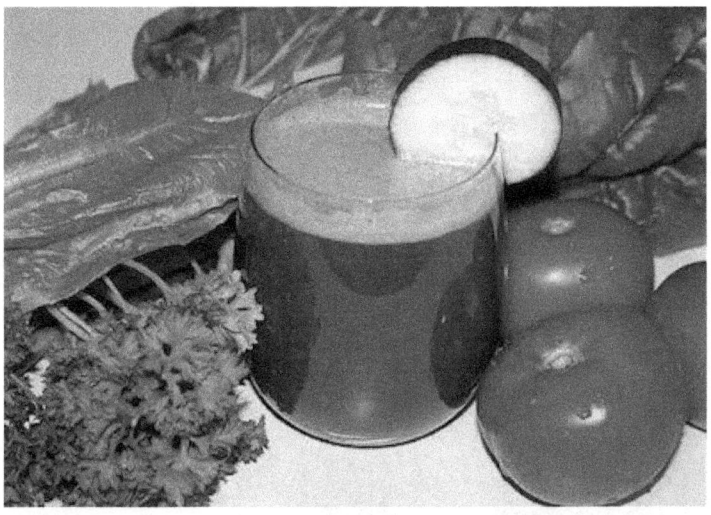

Some juices are all power and punch, others, like this one, are deliciously mellow and pleasant on the palate. Great for when you are after a juice that is nourishing, tasty, refreshing and relaxing to drink.

- 2 tomatoes
- 1 large handful of basil
- 1 large handful of parsley
- 4 stalks of celery
- 2 carrots
- 2 romaine leaves
- 1 cucumber
- ¼ lemon

TIP – If this is just too mild for your mood and your taste buds, add in a couple of radishes for a tasty but fiery kick.

Rooty Tooty

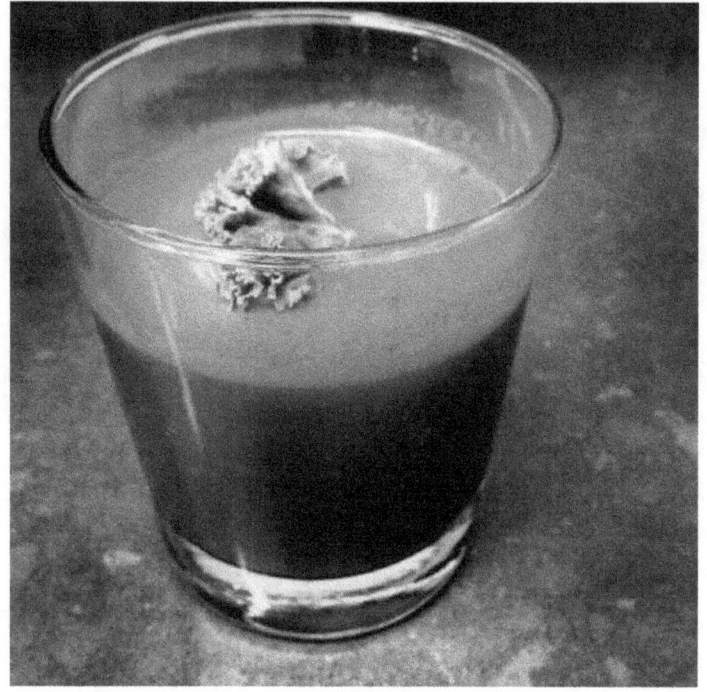

Beetroot and carrots are fantastic root vegetables, ones whose bright colors truly tell the world that they are full of natural goodness. Along with the kale and courgette, this makes a satisfying lunch. Also, courgette is a squash and squashes have been shown to have properties that help prevent colon and lung cancer. No wonder we love it.

- 6 leaves kale
- 1 beetroot
- 1 courgette
- 5 carrots
- A small piece of ginger

TIP – If you want to change up the appearance of your juice today, why not give golden beetroots a go? Their orangey yellow flesh is equally tempting and while they may not be that different nutritionally from good old purple beetroot, it will make a fun change.

Chapter 10

Dinner Juice Recipes

"Dinner time!"

We love those very precious and exciting words, and with good reason. Dinner is often when we enjoy the most delicious, diverse and complex meal of the whole day.

We may have been toiling away in an office or on a building site, or in a hospital… but wherever we work, we are likely to have built up a real appetite.

Dinner saves and soothes and stimulates us. We may sit down with loved ones and chat about our day. We commune.

Accordingly, we realise that dinner is not merely a dietary practicality and nor are these dinner juice recipes.

We have especially sought out juice blends that make an exceptional nutritional impact and boast superb flavours that linger long on the palate.

It may not be a gorgeous three-course meal… but if it were, you would be unlikely to lose any weight!

In fact, a great dinner juice is better than that. It is bursting with three courses of sumptuous flavors in one hit, a superb mixture of vital nutrients, offering complexity and variety, interest and filling soluble fiber, plus it will be low in calories.

Nature's Pizza

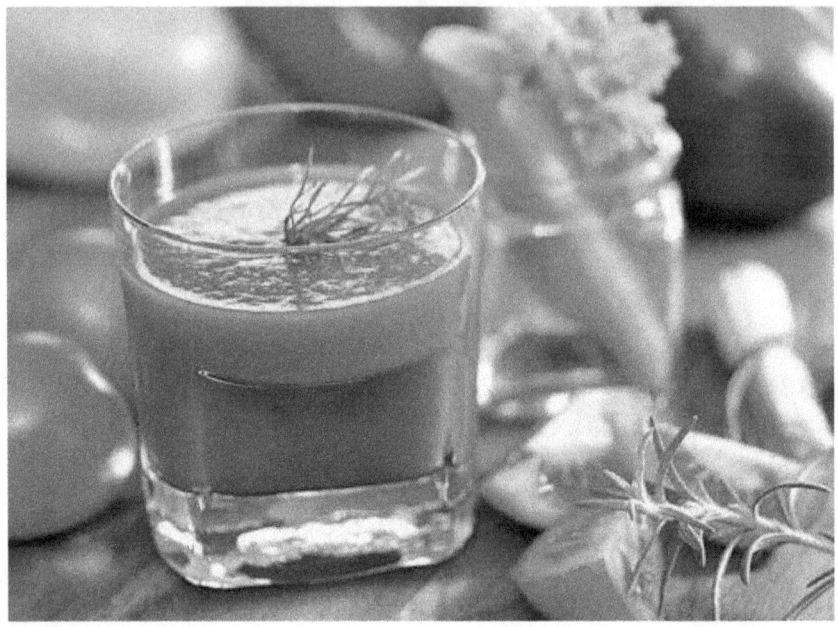

Sometimes on a juice diet what we really want is a nourishing savory hit of flavor for dinner. Happily, this delicious dinner juice is bursting with ripe tomatoes, garlic and onion – think antioxidants, immune system boosters and a whole host of vital nutrients.

- 5 medium ripe tomatoes
- 1 onion
- 3 garlic cloves
- 1 handful of turnip leaves
- 1 handful of spinach
- 1/2 handful of fresh parsley
- 1 jalapeno pepper

TIP – If you are worried about pungent breath from this liquid natural takeaway, simply add more parsley, which freshens breath.

Green Giant

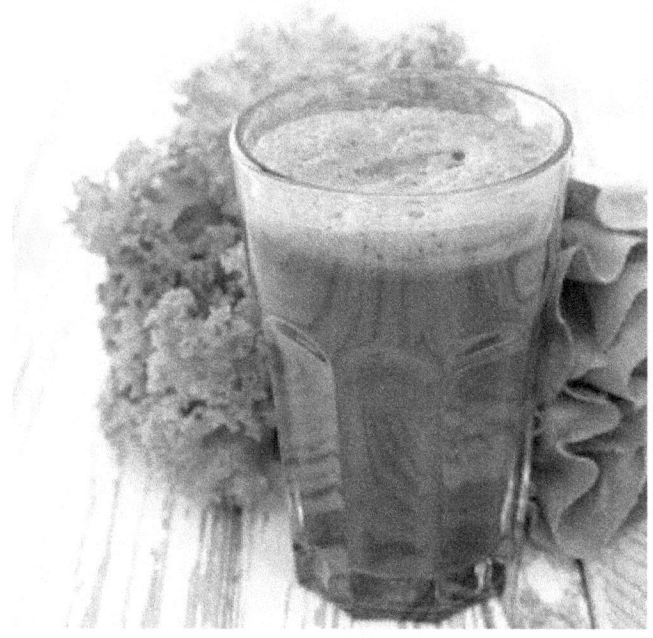

Absolutely everything that goes into this superb juice is bright green and bursting with life. Romaine lettuce added to the mix ensures you will enjoy a healthy dose of Vitamin A amongst many other vitamins and minerals.

- 6 leaves of kale
- 6 leaves of romaine lettuce
- A large handful of spinach
- 2 celery stalks
- 1/2 green bell pepper
- 1 pear
- 1 green apple

TIP – This juice is delicious just as it is but you may wish to season it with a squeeze of lemon, which will sharpen up the flavors and up the levels of Vitamin C.

Royal Flush

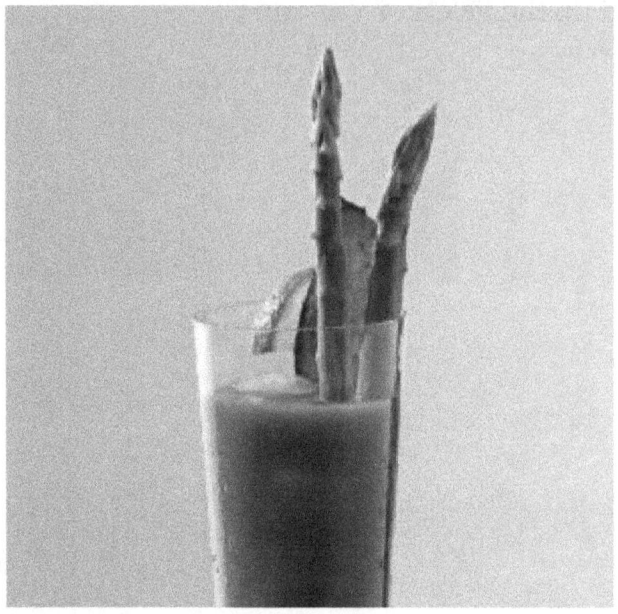

This is a great juice for cleansing your kidneys and flushing through your system. Asparagus is a natural diuretic and has a lovely distinctive taste too.

Very high in Vitamin K, plus it contains folate, vitamin B12, selenium, vitamin B2, vitamin C, vitamin E and much more besides. It must be all those nutrients that have historically given asparagus its aphrodisiac reputation!

- 2 medium tomatoes
- 2 asparagus spears
- 1 cucumber
- ½ lemon

TIP – Try and mix up your tomato varieties to keep things interesting – for example, if you want a sweeter taste, use 10-12 cherry tomatoes instead.

Parsley Power

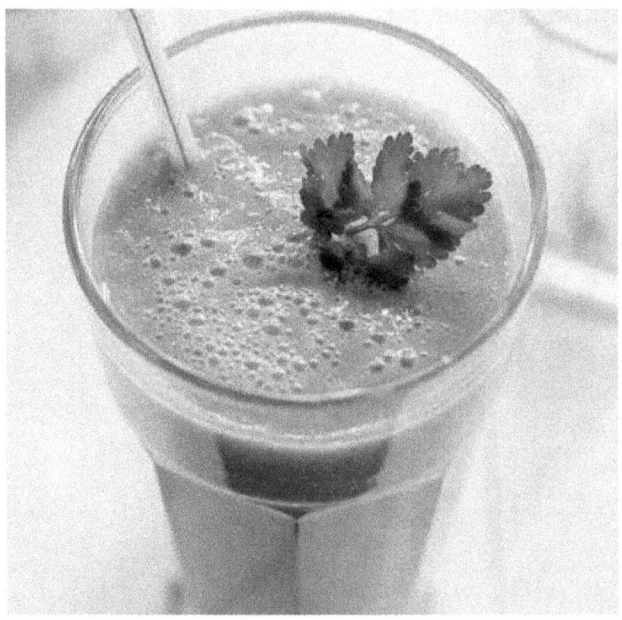

Drink this when you want a satisfying and refreshing boost. This juice is a great energizer and is bursting with nature's best carotenoids, many vitamins and minerals, plus anti-cancer and anti-inflammatory phytonutrients.

- A large handful of parsley
- 2 carrots
- 3 celery stalks
- ½ apple

TIP – This is a good juice to drink before a date – for centuries parsley has been regarded as one of nature's best breath fresheners!

Spinach Sundowner

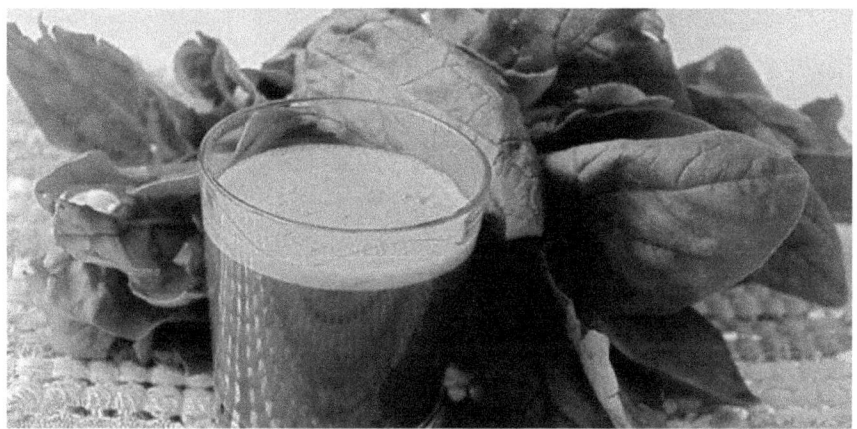

Fill up on this spinach feast for dinner. Spinach is an excellent blood cleanser and is a powerful source of that great nutrient, Vitamin C. The strong savory flavor is sweetened by carrots and apples, upping the mix of fabulous nutrients at the same time.

- 2 large handfuls of spinach
- 1/2 cucumber
- 2 celery stalks
- 3 large carrots
- 1 apple

TIP – Try using a crisp, sweet variety of apple, such as Pink Lady, to give a great flavor balance.

French Dandy

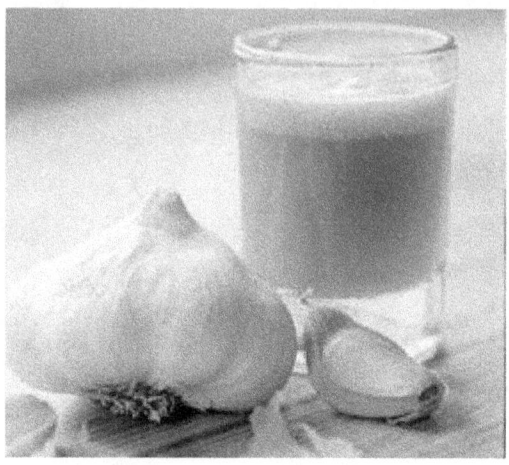

Why the jaunty name for this delicious savory juice? Well the French is in honor of the garlic... and it will leave you feeling fine and Dandy!

Little wonder, since garlic is full of goodness and packed with antioxidants, so great for supporting your immune system. Some studies have also shown that it helps to reduce the fat stores in your body – fantastic news!

Enjoy this juice when you really need an interesting and delicious vegetable dinner juice.

- 2 large handfuls of spinach
- ¼ green cabbage
- ½ cucumber
- 3 carrots
- 1 garlic clove

TIP – If you have had a sweet juice for breakfast, try balancing your fast with this great juice, it has a brilliantly low-calorie load.

Rainbow Celebration

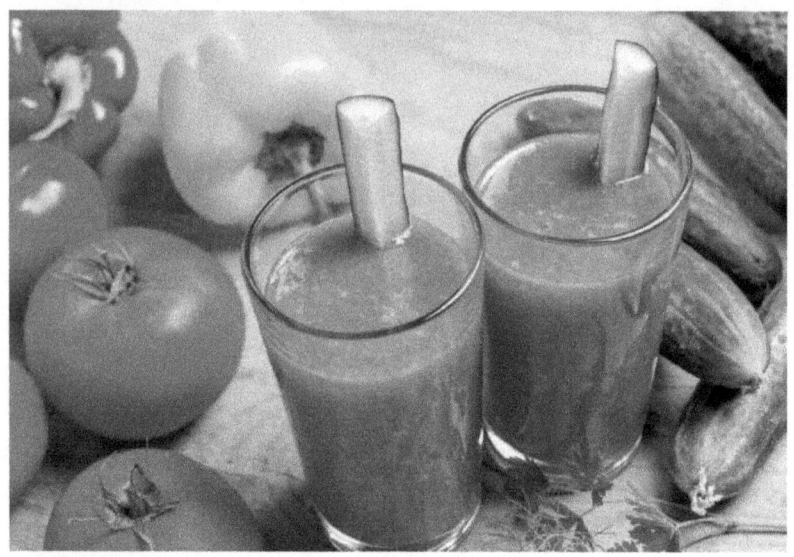

So, what are we celebrating? Your good health, of course! This is an exciting juice to make as it has so many colorful ingredients, which is nature's way of telling you that you are getting a huge variety of nutrients.

There are too many to list here but as a keen juicer you can simply relax and enjoy the fact that you are getting a rainbow boost of goodness for supper.

- 1 red bell pepper
- 2 tomatoes
- 2 medium carrots
- 1 head of romaine lettuce
- 1 cucumber
- 3 celery stalks
- A handful of parsley

- A handful of coriander
- 1 lemon
- A thumb-sized piece of ginger

TIP – This is a great juice to try when you are longing for complex flavors, which can stave off any feelings of hunger. If you want a stronger taste, add in a little spinach too.

Chinese Cracker

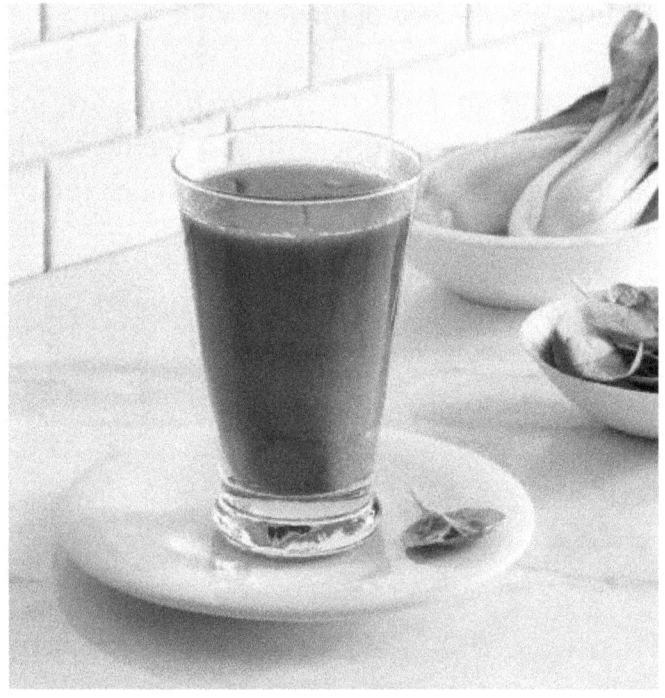

Treat your taste buds to something totally different. Bok Choy, or pak choi, is widely used in oriental cuisine and has a lightly vegetal taste.

It is a good source of Vitamin A, Vitamin C, Vitamin K, Riboflavin, Vitamin B6, Folate, Calcium, Iron, Magnesium, Potassium and Manganese and other nutritional treats.

- ½ bok choy
- 2 celery stalks
- 2 green apples

TIP – If you fancy, give this an added oriental twist by adding in some water chestnuts, which are chock full of Vitamin B6, potassium, copper, riboflavin, and manganese.

Christmas Dinner Juice

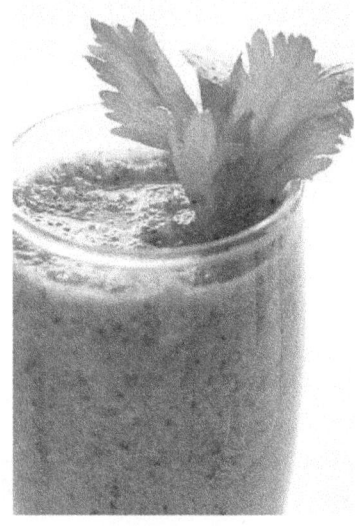

It may be August, but why not? Low-calorie cranberries are excellent for warding off urinary tract infections, plus they boost immunity, lower blood pressure and taste great. Brussels sprouts have unique DNA-protecting properties... whenever you drink this, Merry Christmas!

- 5 large kale leaves
- 3 young Brussels sprouts
- Seeds from 1 pomegranate
- 2 handfuls of fresh cranberries
- A thumb-sized piece of fresh ginger
- 8-10 leaves of fresh mint

TIP – If you find kale to be a very strong taste, throw in an apple to soften and sweeten the taste.

The Souper Dooper

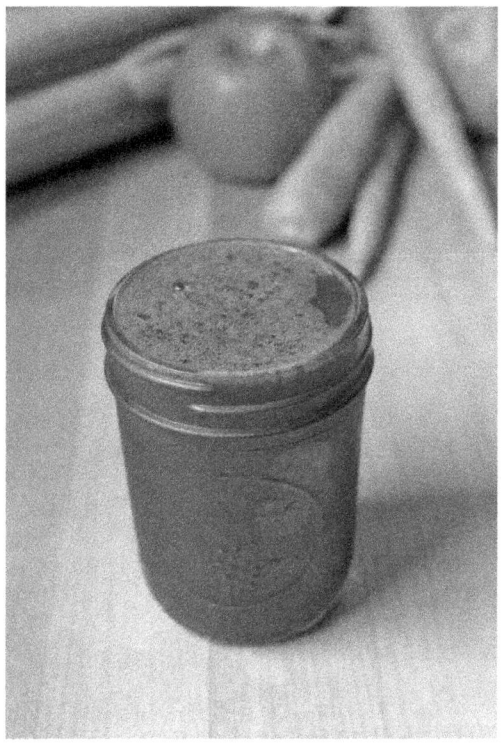

You will love this multi-colored blend of ingredients that gives you all the goodness under the sun. Great for when you feel you want a filling boost that is bursting with vegetable treats.

You must be aware of some of the nutrients in many of these fruit and vegetables from what has been written earlier. But when you juice an outstanding blend like this you can really pat yourself on the back.

Here are just a very few parts of your body that you are supporting, healing or protecting when you drink this juice: beetroot – blood, tomato – heart, carrots – eyes, pears – heart, apples – gut, pineapple – intestines, Brussel sprouts – DNA, broccoli – cells, cauliflower – bladder, rocket – prostate or cervix.

That amazing list just scratches the surface of what all the nutrients in this juice can support. The souper dooper really deserves its great name - sometimes, more is more.

- 1 beetroot
- 1 tomato
- 4 carrots
- 2 pears
- 2 red apples
- 3 thick slices pineapple
- 4 Brussels sprouts
- 6 Broccoli florets
- 4 cauliflower florets
- A handful of rocket leaves

TIP – The nutrient load is incredible and the flavor is wonderful too, but if you really want to take the flavors to the max, toss in a few of your favorite herbs like parsley or basil. Totally delicious!

Spring Green Clean

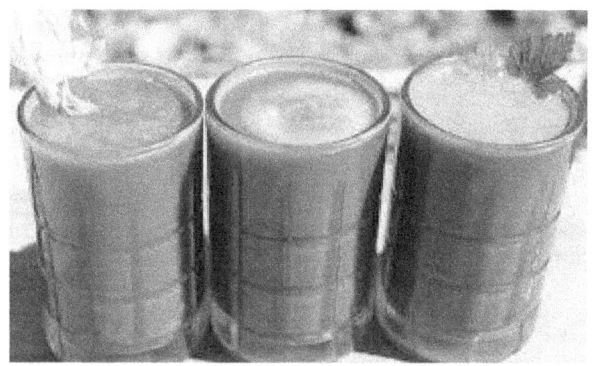

A green juice with a difference. Spring greens are something that we can never eat too much of, yet they remain widely under-used. They contain prodigious amounts of Vitamin C, which is absolutely fantastic for supporting your immune system, plus vitamin K, to build bone strength.

They also contain natural plant chemicals with significant anti-cancer and anti-inflammatory properties, which could help protect against heart disease and stroke. Wow – that's good green stuff!

- 1 cucumber
- 2 Granny Smith apples
- 6 spring green leaves
- 2 celery stalks
- ½ lemon
- 1/8 fennel bulb

TIP – Thanks to a nice balance of flavors, after this juice fast you really could serve this to yourself or others, in a pretty white bowl as a chilled green summer consommé. Sprinkle over some parsley and it will look like the gourmet natural treat it really is.

Rocket Blaster

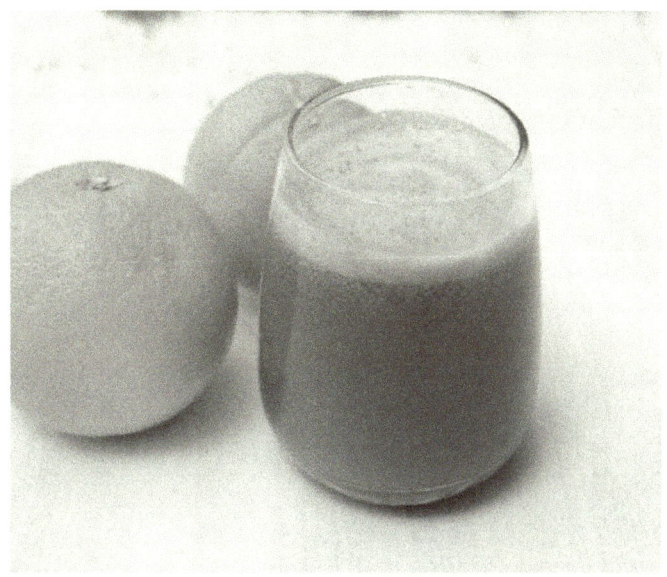

This peppery, minty, orangey blend is full of exciting pep.

No wonder, since rocket gets everything going with its full-on load of vitamins... and how about those phenomenal phytochemicals that can help protect against a range of cancers?

When you blend it with soothing mint, cleansing cucumber and refreshing, energizing orange that is virtually shimmering with Vitamin C... you do really have a rocket blaster of a drink!

- A large handful of rocket
- A handful of mint
- ½ cucumber
- 2 oranges

TIP – For a Persian twist, why not throw in a few pomegranate seeds? They will give you added antioxidant rocket fuel!

Green Genie

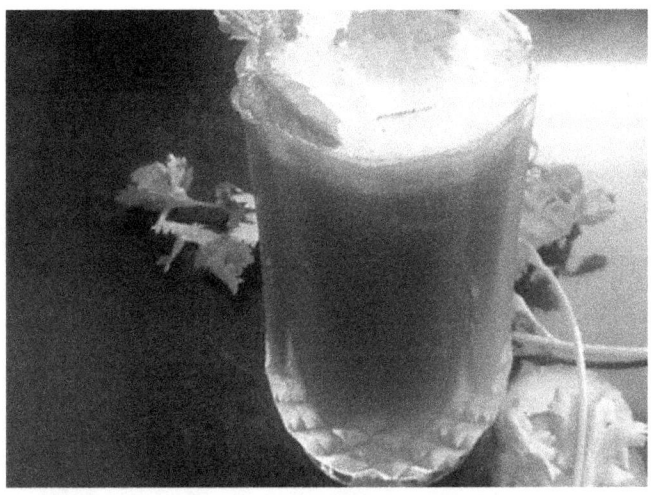

Time to let the genie out of the bottle. Fragrant fresh coriander is frequently thrown into curries and tagines, but as with most plants when they are cooked, some of the goodness is destroyed in the process.

Which is a shame, because there is so much goodness in coriander – so much so that is has been used in the treatment of skin inflammation, high cholesterol, diarrhea, mouth ulcers, anemia; skin, blood and digestive disorders.

Luckily, we are free to enjoy its raw and natural essence in this juice that is full of eastern promise.

- 1 generous handful of coriander
- 2 cucumbers
- 2 Granny Smith apples
- 1 lime

TIP – Do go heavy on the coriander, the star of the show - it has eleven components of essential oils and six types of acids including Vitamin C, minerals and vitamins.

Swiss Delish

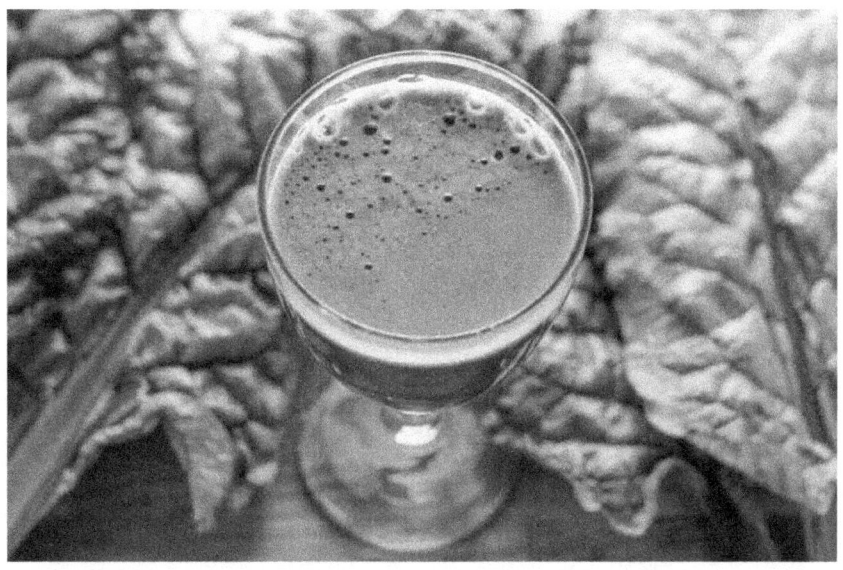

This is a juice that will nourish you at the same time as perking you up nicely. It features some real stars of nutrition and flavor, including the Swiss chard, a leaf that can often get overlooked in everyday recipes.

Swiss chard is not shy when it comes to delivering serious levels of vital nutrients. The plant's leaves contain at least 13 different polyphenol antioxidants, an amazing amount of essential goodness.

- 4 kale leaves
- 3 Swiss chard leaves
- 1 cucumber
- 1 Granny Smith apple
- 1/4 pineapple

TIP - If the pineapple turns out to be not very ripe, add sweetness and cut down on acid by swapping the Granny Smith for a Pink Lady apple, or similar.

Coriander Heartbeat

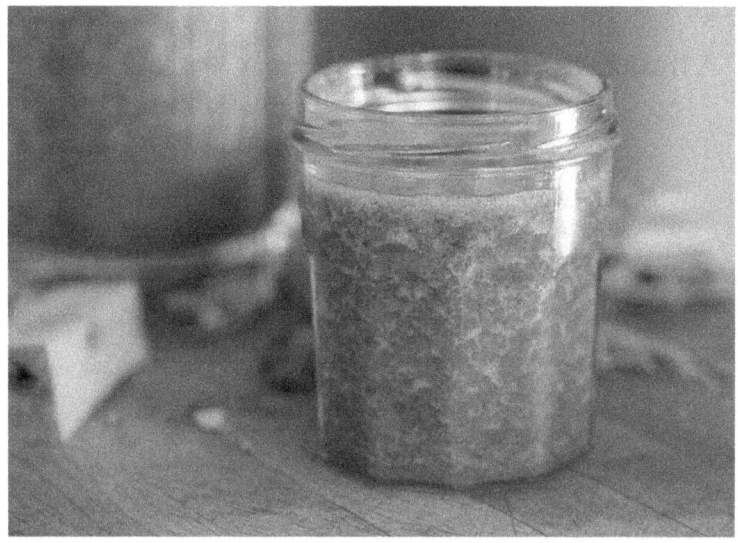

This juice delivers a wealth of delicious and interesting flavor combinations. Beetroot offers earthy sweetness in contrast to ginger and coriander's eastern accent, all lifted by the lemon. But as a detox juice, it delivers even more – antioxidants, Vitamin C, anti-inflammatory phytonutrients.

More specifically, if you choose to follow our tip, the cinnaldehyde in cinnamon helps prevent unwanted clumping of blood platelets. This can be vital to general health as well as helping with specific conditions, since thick sluggish blood causes a long list of diseases.

However, like all great juices, it tastes so good that it is hard to believe it is looking after you so well on top.

- 2 beetroots
- A handful of coriander

- 1 Swiss chard leaf
- 1 lemon
- ½ red apple
- A thumb-sized piece of fresh ginger

TIP – If you fancy a more warming taste, one that feels sweeter without adding any calories at all, try dusting your juice with a little cinnamon. This marvellous spice has a deceptive, subtle taste which complements sweet food whilst not being inherently sweet itself. Remember, cinnamon is not just for Christmas!

Don't forget to share your thoughts on this book by leaving a review on Amazon.com. It takes just a few seconds.

Chapter 11

Snack Juices

Yet another great plus with the 7-Day Weight Loss Juice fast is that you can snack too – on more great juice!

The trick is to listen to your body – if a small burst of a different juice will make it happy then go for it.

These snacks are every bit as nutritious the meals, if a bit smaller and lighter. Try one when you fancy a treat.

Virgin Cucumber Mojito

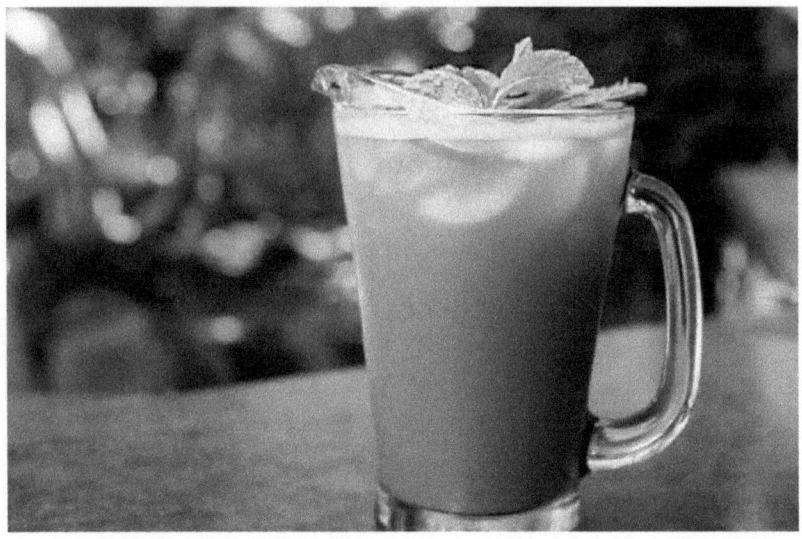

Even a good juicing fan may love the idea of cocktail hour. Happily, this mojito is a virtuous and zingy little number, which tastes delicious.

It is bound to give you a boost when you want a more sophisticated taste. The basil is a lovely flavor touch, plus it is antibacterial and help protects cells.

- 1 cucumber
- 1 green apple
- 1 lime, without zest and pith
- 1 handful of basil leaves
- A good few ice cubes

TIP – This is super-refreshing so don't skimp on the ice and go for a bright tasting apple variety, like Granny Smith.

Granny Smith apples are very high in the flavonoids cyanidin and epicatechin. The combined Vitamin C and flavonoids act as antioxidants, neutralizing harmful free radicals.

Virtuous Virgin Mary

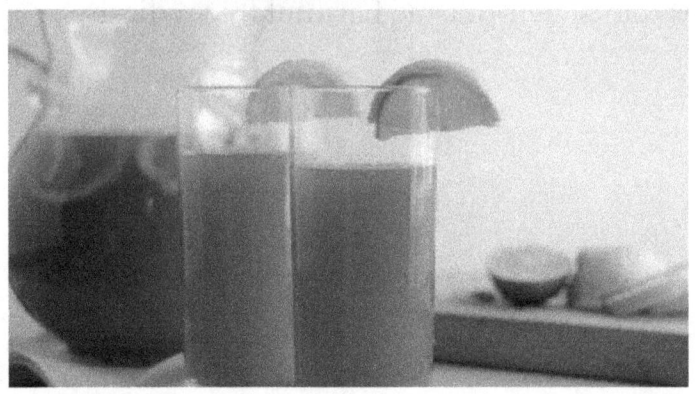

Another great cocktail favorite, detox style. Bright, tasty bursts of ripe tomatoes give a delicious flavor and they are chock-full of lycopene. Lycopene is known specifically to help prevent some cancers, diabetes and heart disease.

It can also boost sperm production in men, prevent age-related macular degeneration and cataracts, prevent skin aging and protect it from the sun, plus it helps prevent osteoporosis. Feel free to add another tomato!

- 2 tomatoes
- 2 green lettuce leaves
- 2 radishes
- 4 parsley sprigs
- 1 celery stalk
- ½ lemon

TIP – If you normally enjoy Bloody Marys with a bit of a hotter kick, add a sliver of red chili to your juice blend.

Fresh Juicy Coleslaw

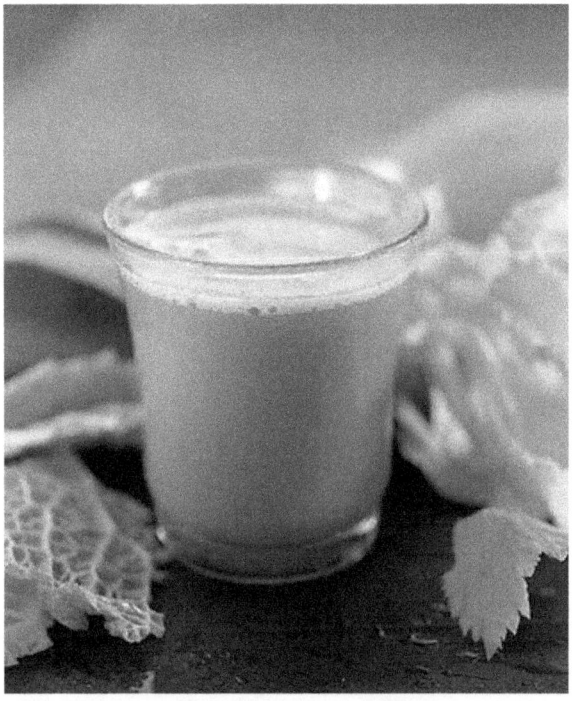

Want a fresh and delicious juice packed with all the goodness of three great ingredients? This blend will ensure you receive lots of cholesterol and cancer-battling cabbage goodness, anti-oxidant beta-carotene, and Vitamin K packed celery and much more besides.

- ¼ green cabbage
- 3 carrots
- 4 celery stalks

TIP – Also makes a great light lunch juice for when you fancy something that reminds you of summer.

Candy Crush

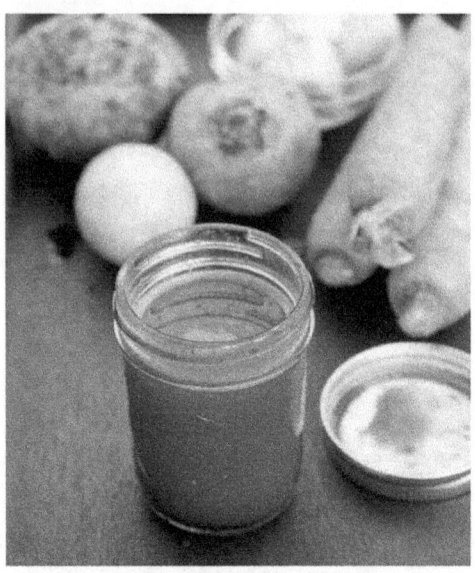

Sweet and delicious with a sour twist, just like some people's favorite candy. But this sweet treat is potent, bursting with nitrates, iron, beta-carotene, Vitamin C, antioxidants and so much more. Beats any 'normal' sweet snack hands down.

- 1 beetroot, untrimmed
- A large handful of spinach
- 3 large carrots
- 1 ruby grapefruit
- ½ pineapple
- ½ lemon

TIP – Enjoy this juice when you need a potent burst of natural sugars and nitrate-charged beetroot power, it's a great pick-me-up.

Watermelon Cooler

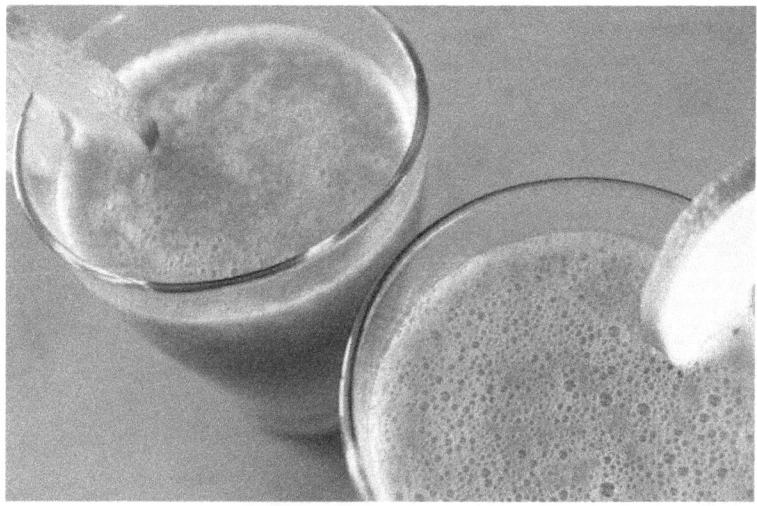

Relish a taste that is reminiscent of a hot day on the beach. This sweet cooling juice is a really lovely treat for when you are flagging and want a natural boost.

Lovely watermelon boasts Vitamins A, B6 and C, lycopene, antioxidants and amino acids, plus a touch of potassium. Superb refreshment!

- 2 cups watermelon flesh
- 1 small lime
- 1 small piece of ginger, about 1cm
- 1 celery stalk

TIP – Don't down this moreish juice all day every day, keep it for an occasional sweet snack. Still, it remains remarkably healthy – and watermelon is 92% water.

Berry Nice

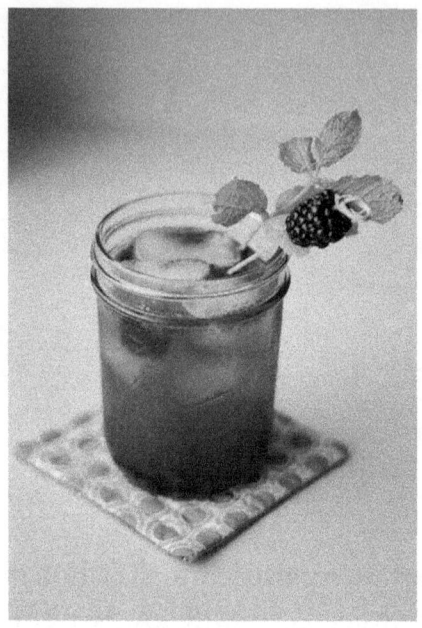

We are sure you have not forgotten that beetroot juice is a powerful cleanser of the blood, and this vegetable is extremely nutritious, being packed with folate, manganese, potassium, iron and Vitamin C.

We have topped up the latter with apples and lovely blackberries, those sweet, sharp, amazing flavor bombs which also happen to contain compounds that may help protect you from heart, brain and cell damage.

- 3 small beetroots
- 2 apples
- A handful of blackberries
- 1/2-inch fresh ginger

TIP – This is a truly delicious juice, but don't choose it as a snack if you have had lots of other juiced fruits that day. This would also make a great breakfast if you wake up feeling lethargic, or want a mood-booster to set you up for your morning.

Discover Scientifically-Proven "Shortcuts" & "Hacks" to Lose Weight FASTER (With Very Little Effort)

For this month only, you can get Linda's best-selling & most popular book absolutely free – *Weight Loss Secrets You NEED to Know.*

Get Your FREE Copy Here:
TopFitnessAdvice.com/Bonus

Discover scientifically-proven tips to help you lose weight faster and easier than ever before. With this book, readers were able to improve their weight loss results and fitness levels. So, it's highly recommended that you get this book, especially while it's free!

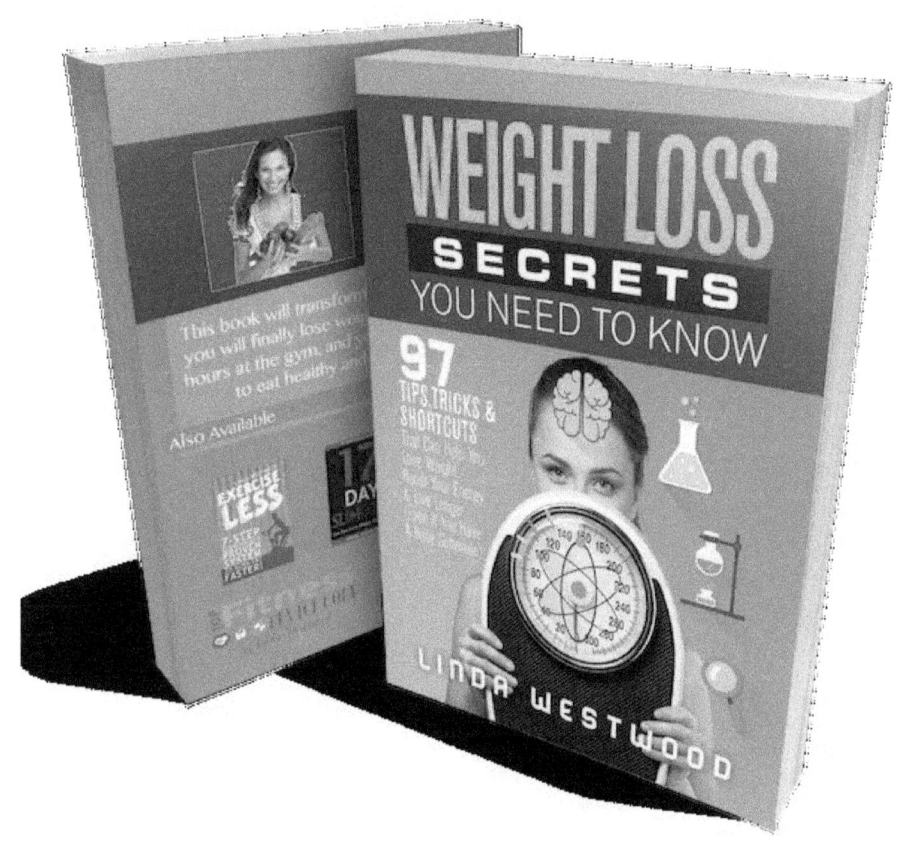

Get Your FREE Copy Here:

TopFitnessAdvice.com/Bonus

Conclusion

So, there you have it, the 7-Day Weight Loss Juice – your super-healthy, totally delicious, ultra-nutritious juice fast.

We hope you have thoroughly enjoyed the experience of undertaking this all-natural weight loss programme especially designed to fast track you to better health.

Now you have successfully completed the juice fast, you will have dropped in weight, turbo-charged your system with the best nutrients that nature has to offer, eliminated toxins, kick-started essential functions like your digestion and metabolism, regenerated old tissue with new cells, hydrated yourself fully, moved your body more, taken high doses of anti-aging antioxidants on board, strengthened your immune system... and much more.

Not at all bad for just 7 days!

Juicing is really just making the most of all the natural gifts contained in every great fruit and vegetable. Powerful, energizing beetroots, antioxidant pomegranate and kale, lycopene-rich tomatoes... these and more deliver perfectly pitched nutrition to our often-neglected bodies.

No longer neglected – after the 7-Day Weight Loss Juice fast you are likely to be feeling absolutely amazing – congratulations!

You will no doubt have noticed these changes for the better yourself and don't be surprised if others start commenting on your clear eyes and glowing skin.

Maybe you will be so kind as to share your juicy new secret with them. Spread the juicing word, or better still let your healthy good looks do the talking!

Now that you have tried out some of these juicing recipes and learned about the many benefits of a juice fast PLUS seen the results for yourself, you have all the tools you need to enjoy longer detox juice fasts, or simply do the 7-Day Weight Loss Juice fast again in future.

Keep healthy, keep moving, and keep juicing. Thanks to simple fresh fruit and vegetables, your future and your health are looking brighter than ever.

Final Words

I would like to thank you for purchasing my book and I hope I have been able to help you and educate you on something new.

If you have enjoyed this book and would like to share your positive thoughts, could you please take 30 seconds of your time to go back and give me a review on my Amazon book page.

I greatly appreciate seeing these reviews because it helps me share my hard work.

You can leave me a review on Amazon.com.

Again, thank you and I wish you all the best!

Enjoying this book?

Check out my other best sellers!

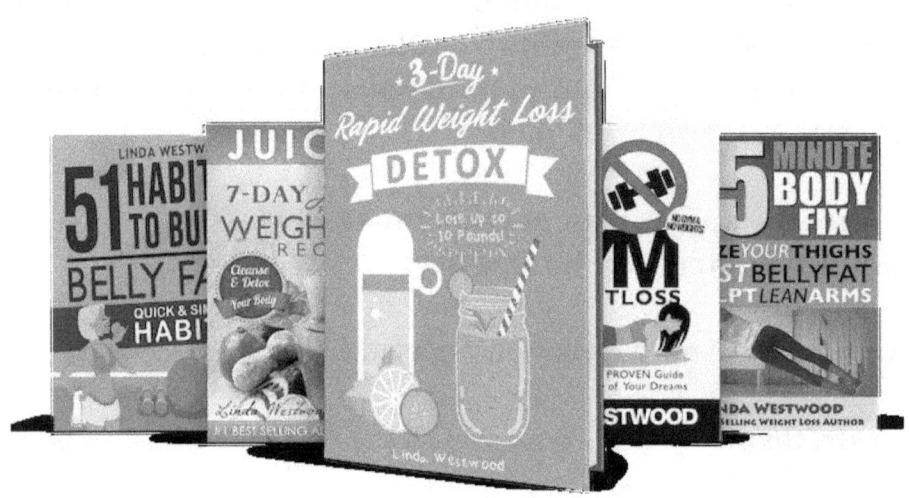

Get your next book on sale here:

TopFitnessAdvice.com/go/books

www.ingramcontent.com/pod-product-compliance
Lightning Source LLC
Chambersburg PA
CBHW031151020426
42333CB00013B/620